ICON BOOKS

Ron Levin
with Gerard Cheshire

The Red Bodyguard

The Amazing Health-Promoting Properties of the Tomato

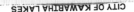

D06731812

Published in the UK in 2008 by Icon Books Ltd,
The Old Dairy, Brook Road, Thriplow, Cambridge SG8 7RG
email: info@iconbooks.co.uk
www.iconbooks.co.uk

Sold in the UK, Europe, South Africa and Asia
by Faber & Faber Ltd, 3 Queen Square,
London WC1N 3AU or their agents

Distributed in the UK, Europe, South Africa and Asia
by TBS Ltd, TBS Distribution Centre, Colchester Road
Frating Green, Colchester CO7 7DW

Published in Australia in 2008
by Allen & Unwin Pty Ltd, PO Box 8500,
83 Alexander Street, Crows Nest, NSW 2065

Distributed in Canada by Penguin Books Canada,
90 Eglinton Avenue East, Suite 700, Toronto,
Ontario M4P 2YE

ISBN: 978-1840468-85-4

The recommendations in *The Red Bodyguard* are based on
extensive scientific research. However, the book is not intended
as a substitute for professional medical or other healthcare
advice. The authors and publishers disclaim, as far as the law
allows, any liability arising directly or indirectly from the use or
misuse of the information contained in this book.

Typesetting by Wayzgoose in 11.5 on 15 pt Foundry Journal

Printed and bound in the UK by Clays of Bungay

Contents

Ron Levin, a Fellow of the Royal Pharmaceutical Society, was managing director of a very successful Johnson & Johnson pharmaceutical company. He subsequently went on to acquire and run many of his own pharmaceutical and healthcare companies, with great success.

Gerard Cheshire is the author of over 100 books including *Collins Gem: Chemical Elements* and the *Science Essentials: Physics* series.

Dedicated to Angela for her patience and encouragement, to Hannah, Esther and Josh for their literary enthusiasm and to all peace lovers everywhere.

Foreword

I went to the market with my brother Jim,
When somebody threw a tomato at him,
Now tomatoes are juicy and don't bruise the skin,
But this one was specially packed in a tin.

Anon.

Tomatoes, along with their close relatives potatoes and tobacco, were brought to Europe from the New World at the beginning of the 16th century. They have played a major role in its economy ever since, though in very different ways. The leaves of the tobacco plant were used as a recreational drug from the time of their discovery until their propensity to produce ill health was recognised some 60 years ago. Tubers of the potato plant are an important supplier of energy and have become such an important part of the diet of northern Europeans that, when the crop failed in Ireland in six successive years from 1845, it produced one of the most famous and far-reaching famines of modern times. The fruit of the tomato plant, on the other hand, has had no such glamorous associations until quite recently when, as Ron Levin reveals so vividly, it emerges as a leading, if not the most, healthful of vegetable foods.

Not only is the tomato in its native uncooked form one of the most palatable, visually attractive and versatile of all our vegetables – which is how the tomato is officially described despite being botanically a fruit – but when cooked it becomes one of our most plentiful sources of dietary anti-oxidants, believed by many to be essential for our continued well-being.

The remarkable story of how the tomato changed from being an ornamental plant grown because of its attractive red fruit into one of the most widely used foods unfolds in the ensuing pages. Ron has, for the first time, brought to public attention the mass of information available in the scientific literature about the dietary virtues of the tomato. Aided by Gerard Cheshire, he has done so in a book written with the lay reader in mind.

Why the story has not been told before is a bit of a mystery, but may have something to do with our familiarity with tomatoes and their association with fast foods such as soups, sauces, ketchup and pizzas, which so many food writers castigate as unhealthy. Ron Levin has assembled the evidence pointing to the value of tomatoes in the prevention of diverse diseases ranging from cancer of the prostate to cardiovascular disease, and presented it in a most convincing and easily readable way. Already one of the world's leading food plants, tomatoes are set to become even more popular, as the quest for vegetables that are rich in flavour and essential nutrients but low in calories gains momentum.

Vincent Marks
Emeritus Professor of Clinical Biochemistry
University of Surrey, Guildford, UK

Why I Wrote This Book

My career was spent in the research-based pharmaceutical industry with a number of companies, each of which was constantly striving to discover, develop and market leading-edge medications, often with marked success. As my personal contribution to that success was negligible, I constantly had the feeling that I was standing in the wings, watching minor miracles unfold. All of these efforts were designed to cure, or at least relieve, existing illnesses and, thank goodness, many achieved their goals.

At the same time I often found myself thinking how wonderful it was that we could keep coming up with new 'wonder drugs' to treat established diseases; but, I thought, what about preventing them in the first place? The training of the medical profession is directed at three aspects of disease:

treatment, treatment and treatment. Little time or attention at medical schools is given to the prevention of disease. So, if not medical doctors, who then should be tackling prevention? Throughout my career, at the back of my mind, there lurked a vague suspicion that a link existed between our state of health and our diet.

During the decade leading to my retirement, at the end of the 20th century, I noted the appearance of several international health surveys carried out by the World Health Organization, the International Cancer Research Fund and others. All found that the frequency of severe chronic diseases such as cancer and heart disease varied, sometimes quite dramatically, between one continent and another, between one region and another, or even between locales within regions. This prompted the challenge of seeking out and identifying the factors that were influencing the variations. From the considerable and detailed data gathering that followed, one conspicuous factor emerged which offered a viable explanation – dietary variation.

Subsequent comparisons of worldwide diets were made to seek out links, if any, that would directly associate individual dietary constituents with specific diseases, both in beneficial and adverse ways. Ultimately, as is well known, a direct link was identified between eating fruits and vegetables and a lower risk of developing major chronic diseases. Conversely, diets high in animal fats were found to be associated with increased risk of heart disease. These links brought about the well-publicised advice to eat five helpings of a combination of fruits and vegetables every day.

The appearance of that recommendation more or less coincided with my retirement. My curiosity as to whether all fruits and vegetables were equal in this regard was aroused. If they were not, which were the principal contributors to lowering the risk of developing major chronic diseases? Moreover, had nature inadvertently created an elixir in edible plants that could help to guard the health of humans? Hence the title of this book.

With time at my disposal, and access to what is probably Europe's leading medical and scientific library at the Royal Society of Medicine in London, I set about my own research project. This involved poring over several hundred studies, which had been carried out by medical and nutritional research centres throughout the world and published between 1980 and 2006. Little by little I discovered that among the vast array of fruits and vegetables, one in particular had become the focus of increasing research attention. It just happened to be popular and cheap to grow across the globe; I couldn't help thinking that serendipity had played its part in this.

Thinking that once the identity of the fruit was made known many might scoff at the suggestion that tomatoes could bring such dramatic health benefits, I decided that the way forward was to provide the scientific evidence. I felt confident that empirical proof, rather than anecdotal evidence, should be enough to convince even the most sceptical. It was certainly more than enough to convince me that tomatoes could make a major contribution to the improved health of populations all over the world. But first they must know about it! So, the aim of this book is to reach people and spread the good news.

CHAPTER 1

The Tomato: Natural History and Human History

Nutritional scientists at the University of California describe the tomato as the single most important fruit or vegetable of Western diets in terms of sourcing vital vitamins and minerals. The human history of tomato cultivation goes back to the Aztec and Inca civilisations of Central and South America. We know that as early as 700 AD a wild form of the tomato was being used as a foodstuff by indigenous tribes. It was probably added to their menus many thousands of years before, when humans first made their way across the isthmus to populate new areas. They would have been nomadic hunter-gatherers experimenting with novel plants and animals to find out which were edible and which were not.

The exact point of origin for the tomato fascinated botanists for centuries. Then a renowned Russian scientist named Nikolai Vavilov (1887–1943) suggested a method of narrowing down the search area. His idea was that the greatest diversity of tomato cultivars, or varieties produced by selective breeding, would mark the region where people had been growing tomato crops for the longest period of time, and so mark the spot where the tomato evolved naturally. The hotspot turned out to be a region of the Peruvian Andes, where a good number of wild species still grow.

Somewhat confusingly, the genus name used for the tomato is either *Solanum* or *Lycopersicon* and the species name is either *esculentum* or *lycopersicum*. This is because classifications have changed over the years. Consequently the full scientific name for the original wild tomato, and all cultivars, can be either *Solanum esculentum*, *Solanum lycopersicum*, *Lycopersicon esculentum* or *Lycopersicon lycopersicum*. All four names are in current use.

The wild tomato found its way into other parts of South America and Central America once it had been improved by selective breeding to become a viable crop. One of the earliest cultivars was the cherry tomato. It seems this variety was the one brought back to Europe by the Spanish conquistadors following their conquest of Mexico, 1519–21, under Hernán Cortès (1485–1547). It is also reckoned that Christopher Columbus (1451–1506) brought tomatoes back with him after his fourth voyage of 1502–04. The cherry tomato is not that far removed from wild stock, as it has fruits that are only slightly enlarged. The Aztecs called it *xitomatl* which translates as 'plump thing with a navel'. Other Central American tribes called it *tomati*, and the Spanish interpretation became *tomate*.

Tomatoes are naturally self-pollinating, therefore their seeds will produce plants closely resembling the parents if they are not selectively cross-pollinated. This has meant that crops derived from the early specimens are still being grown alongside new varieties. Early varieties are described as heirlooms, while later varieties are hybrids or crosses. There are now thousands all told. The fruits vary considerably in form, size and colour; they may be spherical, apple-shaped, plum-shaped, pear-like or pumpkin-like in form. Size may vary from a few grams to several kilograms. The largest on record weighed in at 3.2 kg (7 lb). Ripe tomato colours include black, dark purple, red, pink, orange, yellow, green, white and stripy, but all tomatoes are greenish before they ripen on the vine. The vines themselves may be shrubby or trailing, but they often need help in supporting the weight of their fruits as a result of artificial selection. One particular hybrid, 'Three Sisters', is able to produce three different plants, each with a different type of fruit.

Are tomatoes fruits or vegetables, or both?

Tomatoes are certainly vegetables, since they come from plants, so they are neither animal nor mineral. But there has been a certain amount of controversy about their inclusion as fruits in a commercial context. Botanically speaking tomatoes are the fruits of the plant, just like apples, oranges and bananas, since they contain the seed of the plant. However, the argument arose because they are not sweet to the taste. This meant that the botanically ignorant regarded tomatoes as vegetables just like potatoes and carrots or, indeed, like other savoury fruits such as cucumbers, courgettes, aubergines and peppers.

So it was that in 1893 the tomato's status as a fruit was put to the test in North America by the US Congress of Legislation. This body imposed taxes on imported vegetables but not fruits, even though all fruits are in fact vegetables, but not vice versa. John Nix, a tomato importer, evidently aware of the botanical distinction, challenged the law on the grounds that the tomato, being a fruit, was exempt from taxation.

The case ultimately reached the US Supreme Court for a ruling. Justice Gray provided the outcome of the Court's deliberation. 'Botanically speaking', he wrote, 'tomatoes are a fruit of the vine, just as are cucumbers, squashes, beans and peas. But in the common language of the people ... all these are vegetables like potatoes, carrots and cabbage, which constitutes the principal part of the repast and not, like fruits generally, as a dessert.' Thus, the court rejected the botanical truth. It is worth pointing out that Justice Gray was clearly more ignorant than he should have been for a man in his position, for beans and peas are not fruits, but edible seeds.

The tomato had to earn our trust

Tomato seeds collected by the conquistadors were sent back to Spain where they were duly planted and grown. The Spanish took to eating tomatoes quite readily and they became known as *pome dei Moro* – fruit of the Moors, who were the Arabs occupying the Spanish region of Andalusia until the end of the 15th century. From Spain the tomato spread east along the Mediterranean coast. In France it became known as *pomme d'amour* – apple of love – due to a phonetic interpretation of the Spanish name. Consequently, in France the tomato became regarded as an aphrodisiac. In Italy the tomato was known as *pomo d'oro* (knob of gold) or *mala aurea* (golden apple) because the first cultivars had a golden appearance.

The British and other northern Europeans admired the tomato for its appearance, and initially grew it only for ornamental purposes. The reason was that Renaissance botanists recognised the taxonomic similarity between the tomato plant and related plants with poisonous fruits, such as deadly nightshade, mandrake, henbane and the thorn apple. Naturally, they viewed the tomato fruit with suspicion and advised against eating it, clearly unaware that it was fast becoming part of the Mediterranean diet. The reddish colour of the fruits and pungent smell of the vines didn't do much to encourage tomato consumption either, as they were interpreted as warning signs.

The tomato plant is a member of a large family of plants known as *Solanaceae*, which actually contains many edible species as well as poisonous ones. Edible species include potatoes, chillies, peppers, aubergines, huckleberries, ground cherries and Cape gooseberries. However, none of these had yet been introduced when the tomato arrived on European shores. In addition, unripe tomatoes have a rather bitter taste due to alkaloids that have not been neutralised by the ripening process, so this might have reinforced the idea that tomatoes were toxic.

The alkaloid present in tomatoes is known as tomatine. During ripening the tomatine and green chlorophyll are chemically broken down and turned into other substances, known as carotenoids, by a process known as biosynthesis. Beta-carotene is yellow, while lycopene is red, hence the orangey colour of the ripe fruit. The tomato carotenoids play an important role in this book.

While gaining acceptance as a food in southern Europe, the tomato continued to be regarded as a curiosity in northern Europe and in the US too. It was initially known as the Peruvian apple, and the first scientific name *Lycopersicon* was Latin for 'wolf peach', perhaps alluding to the belief that it was harmful if eaten. Wolves were much feared animals at that time in history.

The first known mention of tomatoes in European literature appeared in a Venetian herbal compendium, written by naturalist Pietro Mattioli (1501–77) and published in 1544. Interestingly he referred to the tomato as both the '*mala aurea'* (golden apple) – and the '*mala insana'* (insane apple), because he too had his suspicions. Nevertheless, he described how it was eaten fried in oil, so perhaps coincidental illnesses were blamed on tomato consumption. It is likely that poorer classes ignored warnings through necessity and found that tomatoes were entirely harmless to eat, thereby proving the scientists wrong.

In 1597 English barber-surgeon John Gerard (1545–1611/12), whose views were influential, declared the fruit to be poisonous in his tome *Gerard's Herbal.* Henry Lyte (1529–1607) wrote of tomato plants being grown in the gardens of English herbalists in his *New Herbal or History of Plants* of 1578. John Parkinson (1567–1650) did the same in his *Botanical Theatre* of 1640.

In 1694 came the first documented example of a tomato recipe in volume II of a cuisine book, *Lo Scalco alla Moderna* (*The Caterer of Modernity*), written by Antonio Latini and published in Naples. The recipe was for Spanish-style tomato sauce flavoured with onions and thyme – a salsa.

The 1700s saw northern European cooks and chefs gradually begin to trust the tomato and experiment with different uses. It had been introduced to North America by 1781, having travelled there the long way via Europe. The third US president Thomas Jefferson (1743–1826) was a keen enthusiast of the new fruit and cultivated it for his own consumption. Nevertheless, the US population generally failed to accept the tomato, just as the northern Europeans had done before them. This was largely because many Americans were European émigrés, so they brought their fears with them and hearsay spread the rumours.

However, fears were eventually allayed altogether when a Colonel Robert Gibbon Johnson (1771–1850) publicly ate tomatoes outside Salem Courthouse, Massachusetts, in September 1820. The spectacle attracted a large crowd, who were convinced he would die horribly. As he didn't even suffer an upset stomach, the crowd was converted on the spot and tomatoes were given public approval once and for all. Johnson chose Salem because tomatoes were strongly associated with witchcraft in that region and he lived there. He had brought the tomato home from abroad in 1808 and wanted to establish a market for his product. It worked!

From that point onwards, tomatoes grew in popularity until they became ubiquitously consumed in Europe and America by the turn of the 20th century. Tomatoes are now well established worldwide as a staple foodstuff. In fact they are the most popular fruit in terms of the tonnage consumed each year. However, they are somewhat divisive fruits; some people love them while others do not, especially in their raw state.

It's the breeding that counts

Tomato vines grown from the seed of the original Mexican stock were found to be rather unreliable. They were vulnerable to pests and diseases, as well as wet and cold conditions. They also produced low yields, and the fruits softened and spoiled too rapidly when ripe. So early tomato growers sought ways of improving the quality and quantity of their crops.

Tomato vines are primarily self-pollinating, which meant that genetic variety wasn't being naturally generated. The solution, therefore, was to cross-pollinate the plants and engineer hybrid vines with new characteristics. The earliest experiments produced the varieties that are now described as heirlooms, because they have been passed down the generations unchanged from that period. They displayed all manner of traits that breeders then utilised to design tomato plants suitable for different climates and uses. Consequently thousands of tomato variations have been produced since the early 16th century.

When breeders cross tomato vines they don't necessarily know what they'll get as a result. The process is a combination of judgement and chance, as breeders hope to combine desired traits into a single variety, but often conjure unexpected results that may or may not be useful. For every success there are many failures. When a good result happens it is then a matter of ensuring that the plant self-pollinates, so that a strain can be developed and a new variety be named.

Processing tomatoes

The first person to process and preserve tomatoes was Charles Nicholas Appert (1749–1841). Tomatoes had traditionally been preserved by sun-drying them, but that only worked in hot countries. So, in Paris in 1796, Appert developed a way of storing tomatoes in glass jars.

The canning of tomatoes was first described in 1847. Prior to 1890, all canning was carried out by hand. Mechanisation was introduced by stages from 1890 and by 1920 mass canning had arrived, thereby stimulating a vast increase in tomato production and consumption. In 1869 a young entrepreneur, Joseph A. Campbell (1840–1900), saw the potential of this process, and found a ready market for his canned tomatoes and subsequent canned soups. 1897 saw the introduction of the first condensed tomato soup.

During the 20th century, rapid progress was made in tomato breeding. The results were increased yields, improved fruit quality, better handling and storage, and improved pest resistance and durability. In addition, there was the development and marketing of a vast range of products containing tomato. Even so, growers still wrestle with the problem of balancing a good looking and pleasant tasting fruit with toughness and bruise resistance. Traditionally fruit is packed and shipped, often thousands of miles, in the firm, green immature stage, either ripening en route or to be ripened following arrival.

Radiation pasteurisation

A significant step forward was the introduction of a process known as radiation pasteurisation from the 1960s onwards. Milk is pasteurised, or partially sterilised, by using heat so that bacteria are killed off, thereby lengthening the shelf-life of the milk. However, heat would cause tomatoes to collapse, so they are pasteurised by other means: radiation. This can be done in one of two ways. The term 'radiation' encompasses both the spectrum of electromagnetic radiation and high-energy particle radiation emission. In the first instance, pulses of coherent ultraviolet light waves from a laser are used to 'shoot' the tomatoes as they pass by, killing bacteria lurking on or in each fruit. In the second instance the tomatoes pass through a stream of gamma radiation particles being emitted from cobalt 60, with the same result.

This practice of irradiating tomatoes prevents them from rotting because the agents that cause decay are destroyed. It therefore prolongs their stability, so that only the introduction of new bacteria will cause the onset of putrefaction. Irradiation has the added benefit of enabling tomato growers to harvest fruits ripe from the vine, instead of picking them while still green. It is worth pointing out that tomatoes do not become radioactive as a result of irradiation, as some people's intuition might conclude. In fact, the only disadvantage is that irradiation seems to halt or, at least, inhibit the continued biosynthesis of the carotenoid lycopene in tomatoes that are still harvested early for long-haul exportation.

GM tomatoes

In the 1980s, the American company Calgene Inc. used biotechnology to modify the gene responsible for the softening of tomatoes. The result was a fruit that ripened on the vine but remained firm enough to withstand handling and shipment. Calgene submitted technical details of its GM (genetically modified) tomato to the US Food and Drug Agency in August 1991, requesting a judgement on its safety. The data was reviewed by FDA scientists who, in May 1994, declared publicly that Calgene's tomato was as safe as tomatoes bred by conventional methods. It became known by the brand name FlavrSavr (pronounced 'flavour-savour') and soon reached the supermarket shelves.

However, the company underestimated public suspicion of biotechnology. Although there was no evidence of danger, consumers demonstrated a marked reluctance to purchase the tomatoes. Consequently, the GM tomato was axed and removed from the shops. This time a public stunt wouldn't have convinced a wary public, because they had it in their minds that harm might come in an insidious way, some time in the future.

As accumulating evidence now points to the health benefits of tomatoes, there is renewed interest in artificially engineering the genes of tomatoes to promote higher and more reliable levels of those chemicals known to be beneficial to human health. Modern GM tomatoes may make a successful comeback if people reason that the scientific benefits outweigh their concerns.

Lycopene

The new and unexpected buzz of enthusiasm associated with tomatoes has arisen due to the perceived health benefits attributed to lycopene, a substance that is present in the ripe fruits. Tomatoes are already the richest source of lycopene, but growers seek to heighten the lycopene percentage in their crops, forecasting increased demand for those varieties.

One of the wild varieties, known as the currant tomato (*Solanum/ Lycopersicon pimpinellifolium*), produces a tiny fruit which, it is claimed, contains as much as 40 times the level of lycopene found in domestic tomatoes. Experimentation with hybridisation has become an active area of research.

Market competition from China, now the world's top tomato producer, has caused prices to fall in recent years. Breeders are therefore seeking ways to add marketable value to their fruits. Lycopene enhancement has become the watchword in tomato breeding circles.

Who is growing tomatoes and who is consuming them?

Currently the top five tomato-producing countries are China, the US, Turkey, Italy and India. Asian countries control 50 per cent of world production, leaving Europe and the Americas with the lion's share of the remainder.

Worldwide, some 35–40 per cent of tomatoes are processed. The marked increase in production and associated consumption that occurred between 1975 and 2004 is illustrated by the following table (*White Book*, 2000). Thereafter world production more or less stabilised, although a percentage increase has been seen in China along with a proportionate decline elsewhere.

Tomatoes are, of course, grown throughout the world and not just in the countries shown in the table. They have become a significant component in the diets of most people globally, not least because of their versatility. People tend to adopt new things when it makes life easier for them and the humble tomato has many culinary uses, which makes it very popular. It is also easy to grow, so that people often cultivate their own fresh tomatoes as well as buying tomato-based products. There are five main types of tomato that have gar-

World Tomato Production in million metric tonnes, approx.

	1995	1999	2000	2001	Calendar years 2002	2003	2004
USA	11.4	12.9	11.4	10.0	11.4	10.0	12.9
Italy	4.3	7.1	7.1	6.4	5.0	5.7	6.4
Turkey	7.1	8.6	8.6	8.6	9.5	9.5	7.1
China	12.8	18.6	22.9	24.3	27.2	28.6	30.0
India	5.0	7.8	7.1	6.4	7.1	6.4	7.1
Egypt	4.3	5.7	6.4	5.7	6.4	6.4	6.4
All others	42.2	47.2	44.3	44.3	47.2	47.2	45.0
Total tonnage	**87.1**	**107.9**	**107.8**	**105.7**	**113.8**	**113.8**	**114.9**

(Data derived from United Nations Food and Agriculture Organization)

nered the most popularity: cherry, plum, pear, standard and beefsteak. Each type comprises a wide range of varieties.

CHAPTER 2

The Free Radical Story

To understand how a food as seemingly banal as the tomato can help prevent and treat extremely serious diseases such as cancer and heart disease, it is necessary to know about a certain phenomenon that occurs as a part of normal human metabolism. The body may be seen as an extremely complex chemical factory in which seemingly infinite numbers of chemical reactions take place throughout our lives. The chemical reactions are essential to maintaining life, but they can generate incomplete molecules that initiate the onset of certain ailments.

The deficient molecules are known as reactive oxygen species (ROS) or free radicals. The definition of a free radical is an uncharged molecule with an unpaired valency electron. Put plainly, it has a 'need' for an electron, which makes it highly reactive with the molecules around it until it has 'stolen' an electron from elsewhere, which doesn't take long.

Naturally, the theft of an electron makes the 'victim' molecule unstable in itself. If that molecule happens to be a DNA (deoxyribonucleic acid) molecule of a cell nucleus then it can cause the genetic coding in that cell to go haywire. In other words, the free radical might act as a mutagen, resulting in uncontrolled cell duplication, which then results in a tumour. Some tumours are benign and localised, but others are aggressive and invasive. Free radicals also cause cells to die off, which is why we show signs of ageing. Our rate of cell regeneration decreases anyway as we become older, so our bodies fight a losing battle against free radical damage until something gives and we die. Combating free radicals therefore helps to reduce the chances of developing disease, and slows down the march towards decrepitude.

Research has shown that varying levels of free radical release make a difference too. Low levels stimulate the growth and differentiation of cells and also protect cells from invading bacteria, but where there are too many for the body to use, the unused free radicals go about corrupting things that they shouldn't – attacking cell membranes and DNA and so on. Other diseases besides cancers can also be initiated by the actions of free radicals. So, the containment of free radicals is an important subject which will be covered in the chapters to come.

The phrase 'free radicals' was devised because they are free – not chemically bound – and they are radical – fundamental and inherent – components in many chemical reactions. Indeed, some free radicals are actually necessary for vital processes in maintaining homeostasis or biological equilibrium within our bodies. They are part of our physiology. So free radicals should not be thought of as harmful per se. But, just as people tend to think of all bacteria as being harmful, so they tend to think of free radicals in the same way. This is especially true now that the phrase has entered the public consciousness in a pejorative sense, in association with the promotion of healthy eating and so-called anti-ageing products.

The very existence of free radicals was unsuspected and contrary to chemical theory until 1900, when Moses Gomberg (1866–1947) identified the first one. He was a member of the academic staff at the University of Michigan when he made his announcement that free radicals exist. His claim was highly contentious and hotly debated in the scientific world for a decade. By 1910, though, his work had been verified by others. In honour of his discovery and its influence on chemistry, the American Chemical Society designated the University of Michigan Chemistry Lecture Theatre, where Gomberg first announced his discovery, a National Historical Chemical Landmark.

Moses Gomberg was a Russian Jew, born in Ukraine. His father, having been accused of anti-Tsarist activity, had been obliged to abandon his home and property and flee with his family to Chicago in 1884. Since neither could speak English, Moses and his father were employed as common labourers at first. By 1886 Moses had learnt sufficient English to apply successfully for a place at the University of Michigan to study chemistry.

Within six years, having gained the letters BSc, MSc and PhD after his name, he was invited to join the university staff. His discovery of free radicals came to be regarded as one of the most important discoveries of the 20th century in organic chemistry and he was widely honoured. He ultimately became president of the American Chemical Society. Even so, ten nominations for him to win the Nobel Prize for Chemistry, between 1915 and 1940, were unsuccessful. The Nobel Prize committee evidently concurred that his discovery was not sufficiently important in relation to other achievements each year his name was put forward. It is true to say that there was a slow-burn reaction to Gomberg's life's work.

I am grateful to the editor of *Chemistry & Industry* for permission to reproduce sections of an article by George B. Kauffman which appeared in the 18 December 2000 edition, pp. 813–4.

CHAPTER 3

Pro-Health Constituents of Tomatoes

This chapter is devoted to listing the constituents present in tomatoes which are already known to be health promoters. Others, believed to be present in minute or trace amounts, may also play a role by enhancing the effectiveness of the principal players.

'Tomatoes are an excellent source of folate [folic acid], vitamins C [ascorbic acid] and E [tocopherol], flavonoids [group of antioxidants] and carotenoids [group of antioxidants] all of which have been associated with cancer protection.'

K.M. Everson and C.E. McQueen, *American Journal of Health-System Pharmacy*, Vol. 61, p. 1562–6, 2004

Carotenoids

This is the collective name for a vast family of natural pigments that are chemically related and synthesised by plants and micro-organisms, but not by mammals, including humans. They are responsible for the bright colours of fruits and vegetables as well as salmon flesh, lobster shells and bird plumage, e.g. that of flamingos.

Several hundred naturally occurring carotenoids, each sharing common structural features, have been identified, of which at least fourteen are found routinely in human tissues. Tomatoes supply nine of these and are the predominant source of seven. Their function within plants is believed to be the absorption of light energy – electromagnetic radiation – for the purpose of photosynthesis. They may also protect plants from excessive exposure to light. Probably the most important carotenoid present in tomatoes is lycopene.

Lycopene

The chemical structure of a carotenoid is a key determinant in its physical and biological function. By virtue of its chemical structure, a lycopene molecule is able to neutralise thirteen free radicals, making it a very potent antioxidant.

Lycopene content varies with the variety of tomato, but the redder the fruit the better. Deep red varieties can contain 50mg of lycopene per 1 kg (2.2 lb), while yellow varieties might yield just 5mg for the same weight. The daily average consumption of lycopene in the UK is 1.1 mg while the recommended amount is nearer 5–8 mg. So clearly the red varieties have the advantage.

The first report suggesting that lycopene was biologically active appeared in 1959. It showed that when mice were given a lycopene-supplemented feed, survival rates and resistance to bacterial infection increased.

Research on the antioxidant qualities of lycopene was sparked by a report in 1969. It demonstrated that the chemical's ability to neutralise free radicals was double that of beta-carotene, itself a powerful antioxidant. Serious study of lycopene as an agent to help prevent major chronic diseases was initiated only in the mid-1990s.

Beta-carotene

Beta-carotene is converted to vitamin A – retinol – following absorption by the body. Although present in low concentrations relative to lycopene, tomatoes still provide enough beta-carotene for the body to synthesise significant amounts of the vitamin. As well as being an antioxidant, vitamin A helps maintain the integrity of skin and tissue lining (including that of the eye) and protects against infection by supporting the immune function.

Other carotenoids or tetraterpenoids

Many scientists believe that lycopene acts cooperatively and perhaps synergistically with one or more of the numerous other potentially beneficial constituents present in tomatoes. Several are also carotenoid antioxidants. They include phytoene, phytofluene, alpha-carotene, lutein, neurosporene and zeaxanthin. They too are essential compounds in human blood and tissues, demonstrating that tomatoes are a very good source of vital nutrition.

Vitamin C

Tomatoes contain approximately 20 mg of vitamin C, or ascorbic acid, per 100g (4 oz). The highest concentration occurs in the seed jelly. By virtue of the quantity and frequency of consumption, tomatoes are third only to oranges and grapefruits in their vitamin C contribution to the diet. A medium-sized tomato provides 50 per cent of the officially recommended daily dose of the vitamin.

Vitamin C is also an excellent antioxidant, which appears to play a role in preventing coronary heart disease by sparing and recharging vitamin E, which is also an antioxidant.

Vitamin E

Tocopherol, or vitamin E, is a fat-soluble anti-oxidant that traps certain free radicals in fatty tissues, especially in cell membranes. There is evidence that a relationship exists between low blood levels of vitamin E and the development of fatty streaks in the coronary arteries. Vitamin E has also been shown to inhibit potentially harmful platelet clumping, to reduce cholesterol oxidation and to contribute to heart disease prevention in several other ways.

Flavonoids

These are antioxidants synthesised in plants. Major food sources are fruits, vegetables, teas, certain chocolates and red wines. They are found in tomato skins, and just beneath in the pericarp layer. Smaller varieties of tomato, with a higher surface area to volume ratio, therefore contain proportionately more. Flavonoids scavenge for free radicals and combine with them, forming inert compounds. The major flavonoids found in tomatoes are quercetin and kaemferol, both possessing high antioxidant properties. While their precise roles remain to be clarified, several epidemiological studies suggest that they too have a preventative role with regard to coronary heart disease. A scientific workshop called 'Flavonoids and Heart Health' in Washington, DC, June 2005, concluded that 'the data presented support the concept that certain flavonoids in the diet could be linked to significant health benefits including heart health'.

Potassium

In trace amounts, potassium is essential to the body. It is used in controlling the body's acid level, in the movement of nutrients across cell membranes, in electrical nerve conduction and in muscle contraction. High blood pressure is known to be an aggravating factor in the onset of coronary heart disease, and potassium lowers blood pressure. Recently, more emphasis has been placed on getting adequate potassium into the diet to help prevent and control high blood pressure, in contrast to sodium (in the form of common salt) which can exacerbate high blood pressure.

Folic acid

High levels of a compound called homocysteine

in the blood are associated with coronary heart disease. Folic acid, or folate, together with vitamins B6 and B12, helps to metabolise and reduce homocysteine levels. For this reason, when the American Heart Association recommended five daily servings of fruits and vegetables, tomatoes were listed as a good source of folic acid.

Dietary fibre

Fibre, otherwise known as roughage, is important in maintaining a healthy digestive system. It can also help to control high cholesterol levels. Fibre is the indigestible part of fruits and vegetables – in other words, the bits that remain undigested as they pass through the gut. They absorb water and bind faecal material together, making it easier to defecate and ensuring that waste residues are not left behind in the intestine.

Compound P3

Research at the Rowett Institute in Aberdeen identified in tomato seed jelly – the gelatinous substance around the seeds – agents that appear to help prevent blood platelets from clumping together. Clumping leads to the formation of blood clots or thromboses. These result in complete or partial blockage of the blood circulation, leading to heart attacks (coronary thromboses) and strokes (cerebral thromboses).

A concentrated extractive, known commercially as 'Fruitflow' and scientifically as 'compound P3', contains these anti-clumping agents. It is patented. It may prove to be helpful to individuals prone to developing circulation blockages, or venous thromboses, that can result in sudden death; long-haul air passengers are a good example. Details of compound P3 research are covered in Chapter Four.

Trace elements

Many chemicals are essential to the running of the body and mind despite being present in extremely small quantities. Compounds of calcium, copper, iron, potassium, sodium, chromium and cobalt are all present in trace amounts in tomatoes. Phosphorus and vitamins B1 (thiamine) and B6 (pyridoxal) are also present.

Other antioxidants

Also present in small quantities are other compounds known to posses antioxidant qualities. They include rutin (sophorin), a nutrient converter, chlorogenic acid, a digestion regulator, and p-courmaric acid, a digestion catalyst.

Not surprisingly, a survey carried out at the University of California at Davis ranked tomatoes as 'the single most important fruit or vegetable in the Western diet' by virtue of their micronutrient content.

Tomatoes are not only nutrient-rich, but they seem to be devoid of any potentially harmful constituents. They contain no saturated fatty acids and their salt levels are also exceedingly low. Their calorific content is low at 14 calories per 100g (4 oz). Relative to other fruits and vegetables, they contain low levels of starch (glucose polymers) and sugars (glucose, sucrose and fructose). In addition, their carbohydrate content is minimal – they have a low glycaemic index. As a tomato is about 95 per cent water, all nutrients have to fit into the remaining 5 per cent.

CHAPTER 4

The Tomato Versus Coronary Heart Disease

Coronary heart disease is the biggest killer in the UK and a major cause of death in the Western world generally. There are approximately 17 million adults aged 40–70 living in England. According to the UK Department of Health, 1.4 million suffer from coronary heart disease and every year some 110,000 die from it. 'Up to 200,000 don't know they have a killer heart condition' read the headline in the *Daily Mail* on 6 July 2007. The figure came from a newly published report by the UK Health Commission.

The stress coronary heart disease brings to each patient and family is significant, and the financial cost to the National Health Service considerable. Efforts to avert just one of case of coronary heart disease are of course worthwhile, but what if 300,000 could be averted? As we shall see from this chapter, that amazing improvement could be achieved if the majority of the population adopted appropriate lifestyles, including the regular weekly consumption of cooked or processed tomatoes.

What is coronary heart disease?

Coronary heart disease is also known as coronary artery disease and ischaemic heart disease. The word 'ischaemia' describes an inadequate blood supply to an organ or other part of the body. In this case the heart is the organ affected. The coronary arteries are narrowed so that the heart struggles to receive enough blood carrying the oxygen and nutrition it needs to remain in good condition. Disease is the end result of a slow but continual accumulation of plaques or fatty streaks, which attach themselves to the inner walls of the coronary arteries. This condition is known as atherosclerosis, because the build-up of fatty material is called atheroma, while sclerosis is the hardening of that material. We know it as 'hardening of the arteries'.

While the symptoms and signs of coronary heart disease are easily recognised in the later stages of the disease, most sufferers show no obvious early signs. For decades the disease progresses slowly, so that the internal diameter of the arteries, the lumen dimension, gradually diminishes. It happens by degrees, so that patients simply put their symptoms down to age. They generally find that they haven't got much energy and tire very easily.

In the later stages of the disease, one or more of these plaques can break away, providing a focus for a blood clot (thrombus or embolus) that can block the blood flow completely, with devastating consequences. The first onset of symptoms is often a sudden heart attack. The condition is known as myocardial infarction and is the most common cause of sudden death.

A number of factors that increase the risk of developing coronary heart disease have been identified. These include high blood pressure, high blood cholesterol, diabetes, unhealthy lifestyle, smoking and poor diet, all of which can be beneficially modified. Factors that, as yet, cannot be modified are genetic factors and the ageing process.

The prevention, or at least slowing, of coronary heart disease development should clearly be encouraged to start as early as possible.

Fortunately dietary measures are now known that can, without doubt, reduce the risk substantially for about one in three potential sufferers. Since the dietary measures are not irksome and, moreover, are beneficial in reducing the risk of other major chronic diseases, their adoption is widely recommended for all, especially those aged 50 years and over.

Prevention of coronary heart disease

Coronary heart disease is the leading cause of death in the USA, especially sudden death. Consequently the US Public Health Service selected the town of Framingham, Massachusetts, as the site for a long-term study of heart disease. Framingham was chosen for the purpose because it had a relatively stable population. This was because the citizens tended not to drift away from the area. Some 5,200 healthy local residents volunteered themselves into the study. The US National Heart Institute, in conjunction with researchers at the Boston University School of Public Health, took charge of the programme. It was set up in 1950 as the Framingham Heart Study.

Initially the study involved some 2,300 men and 2,900 women, from whom dietary, lifestyle and medical history data were to be gathered over a very extensive period. The study, which was still ongoing in 2007, celebrated its 50th anniversary in the year 2000. Some 779 of the original volunteers were still alive and having their routine annual examinations.

The study has been extended twice, initially by adding over 5,000 children who were the offspring of the original volunteers. Subsequently, the second generation of children were included too.

During the second half of the 20th century, nutritional scientists became increasingly aware that a relationship seemed to exist between diet and state of health. Dietary information that had been carefully recorded in the Framingham Heart Study began to be analysed in 1984, and analysis has continued ever since. Much of our present understanding of what influences the development of coronary heart disease has been, and continues to be, gained from the Framingham Heart Study. The Framingham nutrition group marked the 50th anniversary of the study by publishing the key findings and their apparent implications for heart disease prevention. The report stated:

'A better understanding of the influence of food consumption patterns and recognising reliable early diagnostic signs, point to exciting opportunities for the early prevention of coronary heart disease.'

Barbara Millen (Director, Framingham Nutrition Studies) and P.A. Quatromoni, *Journal of Nutrition, Health & Ageing*, Vol. 5, pp. 139–43, 2000

How does coronary heart disease begin?

Before we can prevent coronary heart disease, we must obviously understand what causes it. Until recently research has focused on levels of blood cholesterol and risk of coronary heart disease. More recently a theory called the oxidation hypothesis of atherogenesis, which means the idea that oxidative stress initiates the disease, has come to the fore. Oxidation of soluble fats, borne in the blood, makes them solidify and form the layers known as plaques, which then accumulate to restrict blood flow. The formation of plaques is known as atherogenesis.

The oxidation process occurs when free radicals attack and oxidise vulnerable components of the blood fat molecules. Oxidation is what happens when an electron is involuntarily removed from a molecule thereby destabilising it. If it happens to be a DNA molecule, as it often is, the consequences could be highly undesirable.

When people talk of cholesterol levels they are

referring to the amount of fat being carried in the blood in the form of molecules known as LDLs (low density lipoproteins). Lipoproteins are fat and protein molecules joined as one, and enter the blood when certain foods are digested. As LDLs are essentially the building blocks of plaques, it is necessary to cut down on foods that provide their constituent parts if coronary heart disease is to be avoided.

In 1993 a Dr Joseph L. Witztum provided a plausible account of how the oxidation of LDLs might take place through a sequence of inter-related steps. So the different fats become oxidised first, followed by the proteins. Biologically active molecules, which contribute to the development of coronary heart disease, result. If correct, the oxidation hypothesis of atherogenesis offers scope to frustrate the oxidation process by introducing additional antioxidant support at an early stage. In this way the development of coronary heart disease might be delayed or even prevented.

Can the development of plaques be prevented or inhibited?

If antioxidants can inhibit the oxidation of LDLs, they might offer the prospect of preventing or delaying the formation of plaques. As the development of plaques effectively thickens artery walls, it means that by comparing measurements of the thickness of a patient's artery wall, doctors can monitor his or her health. It follows that one would expect to see little or no change in wall thickness if antioxidants inhibit the oxidation of LDLs. This hypothesis was tested by researchers in Finland. Using a sample of 1,028 men aged 46–64, they looked for a correlation between wall thickness and levels of lycopene in the blood.

As predicted, wall thickness increase was directly proportional to LDL levels. Similarly it was inversely proportional to levels of lycopene. It was interpreted as proof positive that antioxidants do indeed inhibit the oxidation of LDLs.

The Finnish investigators concluded that:

1. Lycopene blood levels can provide researchers with useful information about an individual's previous consumption of tomato-rich food.
2. A tomato-rich diet could help prevent or inhibit plaque formation and its consequences.

In summary, we have a sequence of events which, in simple terms, proceeds as follows:

1. Free radicals attack and oxidise vulnerable molecules in the LDLs to form plaques.
2. Plaques become deposited on the inside walls of the coronary arteries.
3. Deposition of plaques continues over a long period, leading to the thickening of artery walls.
4. The lumens of arteries progressively diminish.
5. The heart muscles become starved of oxygen and nutrients due to restricted blood flow.
6. Plaque breaks away from artery walls causing blood clots.
7. Coronary heart disease concludes with heart attack or stroke.

Oxidation hypothesis – the evidence accumulates

In 1989 the WHO MONICA (MONItoring trends and determinants in CArdiovascular disease) Study was published by the World Health Organization. Its purpose was to compare possible causes of coronary heart disease in populations from 21 countries over a ten-year period.

The report provided some of the first evidence supporting the oxidation hypothesis, for it concluded that death rates from coronary heart disease appeared to be linked to blood levels of the antioxidant vitamin E. The higher the level of the vitamin, the lower the mortality rate. Vitamin E is a well-proven, fat-soluble antioxidant. Studies were soon set up to check whether giving supplements of vitamin E, or beta-carotene, another antioxidant, would provide protection against heart disease. The results were somewhat disappointing.

Evidence from earlier population studies had shown that there appeared to be an association between high fruit consumption and lower frequency of heart and other chronic diseases.

Fruits tend to be rich in antioxidants, especially carotenoids. The carotenoids found most frequently are beta-carotene, lutein, lycopene and zeaxanthin. Studies in which two or more of these antioxidants were present together produced more encouraging results. The implication appeared to be that while beta-carotene and vitamin E are indeed essential antioxidants, for maximum effect they need the support of other constituents present in fruit and vegetables. So the new objective was to identify these other constituents.

Coincidentally, another study was set up by the World Health Organization that came up with some answers. It revealed that there was a marked divide in the prevalence of coronary heart disease between countries in the north of Europe and those in the south. In other words, those populations with a 'Mediterranean' diet had significantly fewer heart attacks and strokes. It indicated that eating plenty of fruits, vegetables, greens, herbs and olive oil made for a healthier lifestyle.

In 1994 an American study showed that a mix of carotenoids was collectively more beneficial than equivalent levels of individual carotenoids in the blood. For the study, 19,000 men aged 40–60 were selected because they all had very high levels of blood cholesterol, but their diets provided differing combinations of carotenoids. Those with a good variety showed significantly less development of coronary heart disease.

Focus on tomatoes and lycopene

In 1995 a study undertaken by Edward Giovannucci at Harvard Medical School, which will be described in Chapter Five, linked tomato consumption with a decreased risk of developing prostate cancer. Consequently, the spotlight was turned to lycopene as an inhibitor of cancers and coronary heart disease.

Another study in 1997, the European Community Multicentre Study on Antioxidants, Myocardial Infarction, and Cancer of the Breast

(EURAMIC), reinforced Giovannucci's work by scrutinising sample groups from ten European countries.

Antioxidant carotenoids are known to be poorly soluble in water but very soluble in oils (fats). The authors of the study therefore presumed that the most likely place for carotenoids to be stored in the body is in the adipose (fatty) tissues.

Accordingly, as a means of assessing their heart patients' recent past consumption of carotenoids, the investigators took a biopsy sample of adipose tissue from each patient immediately following a sudden heart attack. They then compared the levels of the antioxidants alpha- and beta-carotenes, lycopene and vitamin E with that in healthy, but otherwise matched, volunteers. The results showed that higher adipose tissue levels of lycopene and other antioxidants appeared strongly linked with protection from sudden heart attack.

Reports giving added support to the apparent role of tomato lycopene in the prevention of coronary heart disease soon began accumulating in international medical and scientific literature, from numerous research centres in the US, Canada, Europe and Australia.

Researchers based at Bristol University made

precise dietary comparisons between young healthy populations in Bristol, England and Naples, Italy. The influence of diet on each group's blood antioxidant defence status and blood fat oxidation were measured. From this, the researchers concluded that the lower prevalence of coronary heart disease in Naples was due to the stronger antioxidant protection provided by the tomato and olive oil content of the Naples diet.

Swedish researchers, aware that mortality from coronary heart disease was four times higher in nearby Lithuania than in Sweden, sought an explanation. Following investigations they found that:

1. Blood concentrations of the antioxidants beta-carotene, lycopene and vitamin E were much lower in the Lithuanian subjects, and
2. LDLs in the Lithuanian subjects were less resistant to oxidation, making people more prone to disease.

A Finnish group tested the hypothesis that when blood lycopene levels are low, the risk of heart attacks and strokes in middle-aged men is greater. Their study concluded that men with the lowest levels of blood lycopene appeared to have a three-fold risk of suffering a coronary event, when compared with those having the highest lycopene levels. They concluded that, if their findings were subsequently confirmed by other investigators, then it would appear that lycopene from a tomato-rich diet has a role in cardiovascular disease protection.

In the Austrian Stroke Prevention Study, below-average blood levels of lycopene and vitamin E were found to be associated with microangiopathy-related cerebral damage. This is oxygen starvation to parts of the brain caused by plaque build-up in arteries of the head. It is often a precursor to stroke.

Other small but relevant short-term experiments showed that:

1. When healthy adults were given a lycopene-free diet for two weeks, their blood lycopene concentration decreased by 50 per cent, and LDL oxidation increased by 25 per cent.

2. When nineteen healthy adult males and females consumed lycopene (a) from commercial tomato products and (b) from a nutritional supplement, for one week, their blood lycopene increased significantly, whereas oxidation of their blood fat, protein and DNA were reduced beneficially.

3. A laboratory experiment found that lycopene was capable of (a) decreasing cholesterol synthesis by 73 per cent, (b) increasing LDL degradation by 34 per cent, and (c) increasing the removal of cholesterol from the circulation by 40 per cent.

   This mirrors the effect of anti-cholesterol medications, known as statins. Researchers reported that, like statins, lycopene acts as a cholesterol-reducing agent by inhibiting the enzyme HMG-CoA reductase, which is involved with cholesterol synthesis in the liver. The researchers continued by giving 60 mg of lycopene per day to six healthy males for twelve weeks. At the end of this time their LDLs were found to have decreased by 14 per cent. According to German researchers reviewing this study, it equated to a 30–40 per cent reduction in heart attack risk.

4. A European study found that a daily consumption of 330 ml of tomato juice for just two weeks decreased the oxidisability of LDLs by 18 per cent.

In the Rotterdam Study, scientists investigated the suggestion that high blood levels of five major antioxidant carotenoids (alpha-carotene, beta-carotene, lutein, lycopene and zeaxanthin) would decrease the risk of artery plaque formation. Of the five carotenoids, only lycopene showed evidence of reduced plaque formation – it decreased as the lycopene level increased.

In 2003, US researchers published their analysis of the dietary data collected over a period of seven years during the Women's Health Study. The study group comprised 38,000 American nurses and professional women aged 45 or under in 1992, when the study began.

The study concentrated on assessing the influence of four major lycopene sources: raw tomatoes, tomato juice, tomato sauce and tomato purée. Their conclusions were surprising. Women who had consistently consumed seven or more servings of tomato products per week appeared to have reduced their risk of developing heart disease by 30 per cent compared to women who had consumed just one serving per week or less. Risk reduction was even better in those who had consumed ten or more servings a week. Accordingly, they concluded that a high consumption of oil-based tomato products confers cardiovascular benefits.

The same scientists then isolated 483 individuals from the 38,000 who had suffered a coronary event during the previous four years of the study. Their blood lycopene concentrations were compared with those of 483 healthy but otherwise matched women, also from the study. It was found that women with the highest lycopene levels appeared to have reduced their risk of coronary heart disease by 48 per cent. The authors stress that, while the study makes an impressive case for lycopene and tomatoes, other factors, e.g. tomato components other than lycopene, and lifestyle factors, could also have played their parts.

Writing in the medical textbook *Carotenoids and Retinoids: biological actions and human health* (Champaign, IL: ACOS Press, 2005), Doctors Petr and Erdman explained that lycopene and tomatoes could be delaying coronary heart disease development in a variety of ways, such as reducing inflammation, inhibiting cholesterol synthesis and improving immune function.

Manipulating the blood fat constituents

The fat molecules of LDLs can originate from mono-, poly- or fully-saturated fatty acids, which come from our food choices.

Studies at the University of California have shown that fat molecules from monounsaturated sources are more resistant to oxidation. As a result, people with diets high in monounsaturates and low in polyunsaturates are better protected against coronary heart disease. Olive oil is a good source of monounsaturated fatty acid (oleic acid), reflecting the benefits of the Mediterranean diet. Sunflower oil is a good source of polyunsaturated fatty acids, such as linoleic acid. The Jerusalem Nutrition Study obtained similar results, while noting that a blend of both types is necessary for a healthy diet.

Both are far healthier than saturated fats which come mostly from animal flesh.

Platelets hypothesis – the evidence

The discovery, late in the 20th century, of a link between coronary heart disease and poor diet was one of the major events in the history of public health. In particular it highlighted the benefits of eating fruits and vegetables, prompting an international effort to identify the chemicals and processes involved in maintaining good health.

Scientists came to learn about the presence of antioxidants and their apparent role in preventing or delaying the destructive effects of free radicals. But the 'oxidation hypothesis' was not the only line of enquiry opened up by the recognition that fruit and vegetables have positive health-promoting effects. Other researchers made the discovery that the juices of some fruits contain constituents which appeared capable of preventing, or at least reducing, the health risks associated with blood clots.

In the mid-19th century a German anatomist, Max Schultze (1825–74), was examining human blood under a high-powered microscope. He noted, with some surprise, the presence of a vast number of extremely minute disc-shaped objects. He duly described them in a paper published in 1865. Seventeen years later the Italian scientist Giulio Bizzozero (1846–1901), following up on Schultze's work, published the first report revealing that the objects, by then known as platelets, played an important role in blood clotting.

When bleeding occurs, whether internally or externally, the platelets become hyperactive and, by virtue of their sticky surface, they clump together. At the same time, they react with a substance called fibrinogen to form tiny threads. These quickly form a web-like mesh, entrapping blood cells to form clots whose purpose it is to staunch the bleeding. Platelets measure 1.5–3 microns (1,500–3,000 nanometres) in diameter and are therefore invisible to the naked eye. There are 750–2,000 million in each cubic centimetre of blood, which is about a fifth of a teaspoonful. Scabs are blood clots that have dried out at the surface of a wound.

Although clots are necessary to stop bleeding, they are very dangerous when they form within blood vessels. This is because they block the passage of fluid blood, so that regions of the body become starved of oxygen and nutrition. The result is irreparable damage or death. Platelets thus play a significant role in triggering heart attacks, as well as strokes and other circulation problems.

What is more, there is evidence to suggest that plaques conjoin with platelets when they break away from artery walls. They effectively join forces in blocking the lumens of arteries, with disastrous consequences. The antagonism of platelets in this regard is well demonstrated by the fact, borne out by clinical trials, that giving platelet-inhibiting medications to individuals who have survived heart attacks reduces their future risk.

In 1968 aspirin was first reported to possess platelet-inhibiting properties. This prompted several major trials. A comprehensive review of 31 such trials, together involving over 29,000 patients, was published in 1988. That review, which was coordinated at the Department of Medicine at the Radcliffe Infirmary in Oxford concluded that anti-platelet treatment could reduce the risk of repeat heart attacks by 30 per cent. It also found that such treatment could be beneficial for a wide range of patients with a history of blood clotting. While aspirin and other anti-platelet treatments are undoubtedly beneficial, they also bring disadvantages, and therefore the search for better and safer agents continued.

On 1 June 2001, a team of scientists led by Professor Assim Duttaroy and working at the Rowett Nutritional Research Institute in Aberdeen published a laboratory study with surprising revelations. Following up on the earlier discovery that fruits and vegetables can reduce heart disease risk, they were investigating fruit constituents for possible anti-clotting activity. To that end, they tested the juices of seventeen different fruits. Some showed no activity, others showed a distinct but modest effect. One, however, was found to be very potent. It was the juice of the tomato, in which they discovered several platelet-inhibiting chemicals.

These scientists found that fluid could be drawn off, not only from the whole fruit, but also from the pulp and the jelly-like liquid surrounding the seeds. When the three fluids were compared for their efficacy, the one surrounding the seeds proved the most potent in slowing or preventing platelet clumping. It was evident that the substance would be highly beneficial to human patients if it retained its chemical make-up following digestion into the bloodstream. It turned out to be so.

According to the Rowett team, tomato seed liquid extract does not work in the same way as aspirin, but works more comprehensively, without increasing bleeding time and without risk of stomach bleeding or any other undesirable effect. While the identities of the active constituents have not yet been described scientifically, they are known to be water-soluble, to contain adenosine and to exclude lycopene.

A study from Japan has confirmed that clarified liquid drawn from mashed tomatoes impedes blood clotting. Moreover, the Japanese scientists showed that some tomato varieties are more potent than others in this regard, and that for any given variety potency is greatest when the fruits are unripe.

The Rowett laboratory findings were followed up, in cooperation with Norwegian researchers, by testing the tomato seed liquid on human volunteers. Ninety individuals were given either seed liquid or a control supplement (placebo) together with a dose of a substance known to induce platelet clumping. Blood samples drawn from test and control subjects were then examined for evidence of clumping.

Platelet build-up in the test subjects was found to have been reduced by some 20 per cent compared to the controls. Moreover, it took effect within three hours of the very first administered doses. The potential heart health benefits suggested by the laboratory study appeared to be borne out. The human studies, carried out in Scotland and Norway and led by Dr Niamh O'Kennedy, concluded that the seed liquid extract worked by inhibiting the platelet clotting system.

Their work was published in September 2006 in the American Journal of Clinical Nutrition. The importance of the seed liquid extract Fruitflow was recognised by the granting of patent protection in the US. This meant that Provexis, the company that manufactures Fruitflow, was able to enter the £20 billion American heart health market. Patents have also been granted in Europe and Australia and are anticipated in Japan, Canada and other countries. The company is active in the research and development of products based on plant extractives and is reputedly currently investigating banana plantain and broccoli.

Maintaining a healthy blood flow is important for individuals who have high cholesterol, smoke tobacco, drink alcohol in excess or are obese. All of these cause platelets to become 'spiky' and so more prone to clumping, especially in those aged 40 years and over or those subjected to unusually high stress levels.

Overall, it is fair to say that the tomato possesses an armoury of chemical constituents that are enormously beneficial to the well-being of people who are at risk from diseases and disorders relating to both the heart and the circulation of blood.

The European Union Lycocard Heart Project

The seriousness with which nutritionists throughout the world view the prospective role of the tomato as an aid to the prevention of heart disease is well illustrated by the instigation, in June 2006, of the Lycocard Project – 'Lycocard' being a contraction of 'lycopene-cardiac'. It is to be a five-year study, financed to the tune of 5.2 million euros by the EU. The project involves researchers in France, the UK, Italy, Spain and Hungary and is led by Dr Volker Bohm at the Institute of Nutrition of the University of Jena in Germany.

The project is designed specifically to investigate just how the tomato's cardio-protective effect works. Its website, www.lycocard.com, will be regularly filled with ongoing results, all related to tomatoes and the heart. The site is accessible to medical and nutritional scientists, patient organisations and the general public. Dr Bohm is hopeful that 'Lycocard will lead to what everyone seeks – a reason to eat something which is both delicious and good for you'.

Because studies will be performed with healthy subjects, the results are expected to help create guidelines for early heart disease prevention. For example, the project anticipates that eating five fruit or vegetable portions every day, including tomato, could be one such guideline. Because close links exist between oxidative stress, inflammation, obesity and heart disease, the effects of diets enriched with tomato products, and therefore containing high levels of lycopene, will be assessed in obese patients.

Lycocard undertakes to provide the medical community and patient groups with the results of their research and their implications for helping to maintain healthy hearts. The information is expected to lead to the development of healthy new foods based on tomatoes, and high consumer demand for such health-related tomato products. Lycocard believes it will help improve the health of European and other consumers, thereby reducing the cost of running health services.

Summary

In spite of the scientific evidence presented, whether or not the oxidation and blood clotting hypotheses are the definitive explanations for the development of heart disease remains to be proven. However the positive protective roles of the constituents in fruits and vegetables, combined with a healthy lifestyle, remain unchallenged. Tomatoes and their products, by virtue of their exceptionally wide spectrum of antioxidants and other protective components, are undoubtedly the fruit (or vegetable if you prefer) of choice. Fortunately, the tomato is widely cultivated and has become one of the world's major crops. It is almost universally available and relatively inexpensive.

CHAPTER 5

The Tomato Versus Prostate Cancer

This chapter is devoted to prostate cancer because, along with coronary heart disease, it has been the most intensively researched ailment to date in relation to tomato and lycopene consumption. Tomatoes could also play a useful role with respect to other cancers, as we shall see in Chapter Seven.

In 1981, following years of careful study, two British epidemiologists and their colleagues published a far-sighted prophecy based on a combination of scientific evidence and intuition. Within 25 years, they predicted, the scientific community would have come up with the goods to back their suggestion that plant chemicals would be found to have anti-carcinogenic properties:

'There is growing evidence that retinoid and perhaps carotenoids may be anti-carcinogenic ... possible mechanisms include protection ... by enhancing some immunological function or by quenching singlet oxygen and trapping free radicals ... which may be generated as a by-product in many normal metabolic processes ... It seems probable a few truly protective agents await discovery among a dozen or so dietary factors of current interest to the research community.'

R. Peto, R. Doll, J.D. Buckley and A.B. Sporn,
Nature, Vol. 290, p. 201, 1981

Prostate cancer has been increasing worldwide, at a rate of 3 per cent per year, for at least 25 years. Some, but not all, recorded cases are due to better and much earlier detection resulting from the introduction of PSA (prostate specific antigen) blood tests. It is known that the risk of developing the disease increases sharply with age beyond 60, and is said to be 130 times greater at age 75–79 years than at age 45–49.

What is prostate cancer?

The prostate gland is walnut-sized and lies between the bladder and the root of the penis.

The urethra, the tube that carries urine from the bladder, passes through the centre of the prostate. During arousal, the urethra carries the fluid part of semen from the prostate gland, where it is produced. Cancers usually arise in the rear portion of the gland itself, near to the rectum.

Cancer arises when cells of the prostate begin to grow uncontrollably, creating small tumours. Tumour cells outlive normal cells and continue to form new abnormal cells. In most cases prostate cancer is slow growing, and it may take several years, perhaps even one or two decades, to become large enough to produce detectable symptoms. This is generally good news, as it provides opportunity for steps to be taken to stop or slow the growth.

Although treatment has improved considerably in recent years, the death toll is still high. Preventative strategies have recently moved to the forefront, and nutritional strategies for improving prevention and treatment are becoming more prominent. While some of the factors that increase an individual's risk of developing prostate cancer, such as age, ethnic origin and family history, are unchangeable, there are others that, when tackled appropriately, appear to reduce the risk quite significantly.

This chapter will follow the path leading to the realisation and virtual acknowledgment that the consumption of tomatoes can help prevent or inhibit the development of prostate cancer. Some of the important milestones on the way will be identified.

Can prostate cancer be prevented or inhibited?

Between 1978 and 1982 a large number of studies, monitoring both large and small populations, were published, showing that people who consumed higher quantities of vegetables appeared to develop cancer less frequently than those who regularly ate lower quantities.

Closer examination of the data revealed that it was the yellow and green vegetables that seemed to be providing the beneficial effects. A possible explanation for the difference between the effects of the vegetables was, at the time, thought to be related to their carotenoid content. This was probably because, in 1983, Peto and his colleagues at Oxford had published an extensive review which concluded that members of the carotenoid family appeared to help prevent cancer.

In 1976 medical and nutritional scientists at the Harvard Medical School Centre for Cancer

Prevention in Boston, USA set up a number of studies designed to investigate whether or not any relationship could be found between diet and cancer. Their first study involved some 13,000 Boston area residents, aged 66 years and over, who were free from cancer at the outset. Normal dietary intake for each of 41 food items was recorded for each individual; they were then monitored frequently and regularly for almost five years. At the end of this time the investigators compared the diets of the survivors with the diets of those who had died from cancer during the survey period. The diets of those who had died were found to have contained much lower quantities of strawberries and tomatoes. Subsequent studies failed to confirm the effect of strawberries but, as we shall see, with tomatoes it was a quite different story.

In the mid-1970s, scientists at Johns Hopkins University in Baltimore, USA set out to find whether there was any link between the intake of six specific nutrients believed to assist in the prevention of bladder cancer and the subsequent development of the disease. Blood was collected from some 26,000 volunteers who had donated it specifically for use in cancer research. Over the following eleven years, 35 new cases of bladder cancer were diagnosed among the volunteers. The blood samples, which had been collected in 1975 and stored throughout the eleven years at minus 70 °C to maintain their stability, were then examined and analysed.

Blood samples from the volunteers who had developed bladder cancer were compared with those of matched volunteers who remained cancer free. The analysis showed that blood levels of two of the six specific nutrients had been significantly lower in the volunteers who had subsequently developed cancer. These were selenium and lycopene. Studies, which will be discussed in Chapter Seven, found that patients with several other forms of cancer also had low blood levels of lycopene.

Earlier surveys carried out among Seventh Day Adventists had suggested a low risk of prostate cancer among this community. To investigate this further, 14,000 men in the community completed a lifestyle questionnaire in 1976. It included detailed information about their diets. They were then monitored over six years for the appearance of any forms of cancer. The investigating team concluded that 'unidentified anti-cancer constituents' present in their diets appeared to be exerting a protective effect. This effect, they believed, related to intake of legumes, dried fruits and/or tomatoes.

One of the first, if not the very first, studies to report a beneficial health effect from tomato consumption came from northern Iran, where cancer of the gullet is very prevalent. Weekly tomato consumption was reported to have reduced that cancer risk by a remarkable 40 per cent.

Another of the Harvard studies, this time set up in 1986, was to draw unexpectedly dramatic conclusions nine years later. Known as the Health Professionals Follow-up Study (HPFS) it recruited some 48,000 men, all health professionals (dentists, pharmacists, osteopaths, veterinarians, etc.) and aged 40–75 years. All were free from symptoms of heart disease and cancer. Detailed food questionnaires were collected from each of the volunteers at regular intervals. Within nine years, 812 new cases of prostate cancer had been detected in the group.

The intake of 46 foods – fruits, vegetables and related products – consumed by the prostate cancer patients was compared with that of matched volunteers who had remained free from disease. Of the 46 food items monitored, only four were found to be significantly related to a lower risk of prostate cancer. These were tomato sauce, fresh tomatoes, tomato juice and tomato purée. Men who had regularly eaten ten or more helpings per week had reduced their risk of developing prostate cancer during the nine-year period by no less than 30 per cent, as compared to those who consistently consumed one helping or less.

At least fourteen carotenoids are present in human blood and tissues. Predominant among these are alpha-carotene and beta-carotene, lutein, betacryptoxanthin and lycopene. By checking food constituent reference tables, the Harvard scientists were able to calculate the quantities of each of these five principal carotenoids present in the diets of the 48,000 men. Of the five, only one was found to be clearly related to the reduced risk of prostate cancer. It was lycopene, the red pigment that gives ripe tomatoes their colour. Tomatoes and, to a much lesser extent, watermelon and pink grapefruit, are the primary sources of lycopene in Western diets.

Surprisingly, tomato sauce for pasta appeared to be more effective than raw tomato. Tomato sauce for pasta is produced by cooking ripe tomatoes in a mixture containing oil, usually olive oil. This Harvard study was the first to suggest a role for tomato sauce in prostate cancer prevention. The Harvard team noted that high tomato consumption is a feature of the diet in Italy and Greece, Mediterranean countries where mortality from prostate cancer is significantly lower.

The source and quality of the Harvard tomato study, which was published in 1995, prompted considerable interest among nutritional research scientists in the USA, Canada, the UK, continental Europe, Israel, India, China, Asia, Russia and Australasia, from whence a vast number of published studies have subsequently emerged.

Running alongside the HPFS, the Harvard Group had, in 1982, previously set up another long-term study. This time it involved over 22,000 male US physicians, who were aged 40–84 years and free from cancer. Blood measurements were taken at the outset, which included levels of the five principal carotenoids. After thirteen years, the diets of 578 subjects who had been diagnosed with prostate cancer and 1,294 non-cancerous matched control subjects were analysed and compared. Of the five carotenoids, once again lycopene was the only one consistently associated with a reduced risk of prostate cancer, and once again the strongest protective effect was seen in men who had frequently consumed cooked tomato products, especially tomato sauce.

Oxidation – is this where it begins?

An antioxidant was defined in 1989 as 'a substance which when present in low concentration, as compared with that of the oxidisable substance, (e.g. cholesterol), significantly delays or inhibits its oxidation'. It therefore follows that, where a disease is initiated or enhanced by oxidation within the body's cells or tissues, the presence or introduction of an antioxidant or combination of antioxidants could possibly protect the cells or tissues, thereby preventing or delaying the development of disease.

This hypothesis is central to an understanding of how antioxidants might contribute to good health preservation and disease prevention. Free radicals can cause oxidative damage to cell membranes and DNA, thereby triggering uncontrolled cellular growth – cancers. The presence, in adequate concentrations, of powerful antioxidants such as lycopene could conceivably quench these radicals instantly as they arise.

Scientists at the University of Toronto in Canada, prompted by the Harvard study, investigated the ease with which lycopene is absorbed into the bloodstream following tomato consumption. Tomato sauce, tomato purée and tomato juice were given at intervals to healthy volunteers. Each time, the concentration of lycopene in the blood was measured before and after. All three forms led to significant increases in lycopene blood concentration. Moreover, the antioxidant capacity of the blood and antioxidant protection of the blood DNA, protein and fat content were all enhanced.

The evidence builds up

Professors Edward Giovannucci of Harvard and Steve Clinton of Ohio are two leading contemporary investigators into tomato, lycopene and prostate cancer prevention. Writing in 1998, they cautioned against the assumption that lycopene, or products rich in lycopene, are necessarily directly responsible for the reported beneficial effects. Perhaps, they argued, lycopene and tomato products are simply routinely present alongside the real active substance. Or they stimulate a process within the body, e.g. hormone status or immune function, which actually does the job. Perhaps substances present in tomatoes other than lycopene play a vital role.

If lycopene is to have a direct effect on prostate cancer cells, they wrote, it must be detectable in prostate tissues. Their subsequent studies on the pattern and concentrations of carotenoids in the human prostate showed not only that lycopene was indeed present in the majority of prostate glands, but that it was at a higher concentration there than in the blood.

In 1999, Giovannucci reviewed 72 population and clinical studies into tomatoes, lycopene and prostate cancer prevention which had already been published in the international scientific literature. Of these, he found that 57 had found a reduced risk of several different cancers; in 35 of these, the findings were statistically validated. The strongest evidence related to cancers of the prostate, lung and stomach, although the data suggested benefits in other cancers too.

As fifteen of the 72 published studies had failed to show a benefit, Giovannucci returned to the subject in 2002 after considering possible reasons for their failure. He noted that studies initiated before 1995 had been unaware of the importance of tomatoes, so they were largely overlooked. Also, different tomato products vary in their concentrations of lycopene. While the beneficial effects from tomato sauce are substantial, those from fresh tomatoes and tomato purée are moderate, while those of tomato juice are even less significant. The reasons for this will be explained in Chapter Six.

In 1999, Giovannucci wrote that 'based on the consistency of the evidence, the association of tomato and tomato products with reduced prostate cancer risk is direct'.

Mortality from prostate cancer in Greece is well below that in the USA, the UK and northern Europe. Seeking a possible explanation, Greek researchers compared the diet of 320 prostate cancer patients with that of a similar number of matched control volunteers. Tomato consumption was found to have been much higher among the cancer-free individuals.

The Sloan-Kettering Institute in New York is a universally recognised centre of excellence for cancer research and treatment. Not surprisingly, its scientists, fascinated by the reports describing an apparent role for tomatoes in cancer prevention, set about checking these claims via their own studies. They compared the carotenoid levels in the blood of prostate cancer patients and matched cancer-free control subjects. They too found that lycopene and other carotenoid concentrations were much higher in the healthy control subjects. They concluded that their study had confirmed previous reports and that, moreover, other closely related tomato carotenoids – lutein, zeaxanthin and betacryptoxanthin – together with vitamin E, probably also play roles. This subsequently proved to be correct.

Some of the nutritional and medical scientists who had been investigating tomatoes, lycopene and cancer prevention pooled their findings at a seminar, sponsored by Heinz, in March 2000. Medical oncologist Dr Omer Kucuk described one of the first studies carried out in prostate cancer patients. In his study, a group who were due to undergo surgery for diseased prostate removal were given a lycopene preparation daily for three weeks before surgery. When their prostate glands were compared to those of the patients who had not taken supplements, they showed smaller and more localised tumours. Microscopic growth of the cancers had decreased and PSA (prostate specific antigen) indicator had decreased by 18 per cent, leading Kucuk to speculate that tomato lycopene may have a role in the orthodox treatment of prostate cancer as well as in its prevention. This view was later shared by other researchers.

Kucuk is now undertaking a large trial among advanced prostate cancer patients. A similar pre-surgery study was presented at the March 2000 symposium by Phyllis Bowen and colleagues. Every day for three weeks, they gave men due to undergo prostate removal a tomato sauce supplement containing a 30 mg dose of lycopene. Post-surgical blood and prostate tissue analyses revealed that lycopene levels had increased while prostate cell DNA damage had decreased. This preliminary study is being followed up by a major trial from which the scientists believe that 'if [conclusions are] consistent with our preliminary findings this will make a case for adding lycopene to conventional prostate cancer treatments'.

John Weisburger, Director of the American Health Foundation, concluded the symposium by raising three major issues:

1. Why do people in the Mediterranean region have a much lower risk of heart disease and nutrition-linked cancers? Is it because an important component of their diet is tomatoes cooked together with olive oil? Olive oil contains vitamin E.
2. Do free radicals, which are produced in the body during normal metabolism and inhaled from tobacco smoke or air pollution, attack the DNA in genes, leading to mutations that mark the initiation of all types of cancer?
3. Modern medical science expects disease-preventing agents to be assessed using classical clinical trial methods, as are used for the treat-

ment of disease, without which many doctors are unwilling to accept the claims. For disease prevention, as distinct from treatment, such studies would have to be lengthy and include very large numbers of people who are perfectly healthy at the outset of the study. Can we accept the idea that classical clinical trial requirements are simply not practicable, and that other methods must be found?

This latter view was supported by Clinton's group, who agreed that such studies could take decades, with attendant prohibitive costs. Instead, they recommended that results and conclusions arrived at by a combination of population studies, clinical studies in patients, animal models and testing against isolated human prostate cancer cells would, together, bring definitive conclusions in a much shorter time.

A progress report, published in 2002 by Phyllis Bowen and her deeply involved research group, concluded that 'lycopene, or lycopene in combination with other substances in tomatoes, may be a viable bioactive compound for use in the prevention of some cancers'. Moreover, they added that, with more than 100 human studies published by 2002, the time had come for a thorough investigation of lycopene, both as a preventive and as an addition to conventional treatments.

Coincidentally, the same conclusion was drawn by Giovannucci and Clinton, who updated their combined view to the following:

1. That lycopene may prove to be most effective against advanced and aggressive prostate cancer, and
2. That tomato constituents other than lycopene probably contribute to the effect.

In order to reduce the risk of prostate cancer, other cancers and other major chronic diseases, for example heart disease, they recommended that the general population consume one serving of tomato products daily, or a least five servings per week, as part of an overall healthy diet.

At the international research conference Food, Nutrition and Cancer, held in Washington, DC in July 2004, new data was presented from the previously mentioned HPFS study, which had now extended to twelve years. The earlier conclusion, that regular consumption of tomato products is associated with a reduced risk of prostate cancer, was again confirmed. Furthermore, just two servings a week of tomato sauce (which appears to be the most effective form) were found to be enough to produce a 23 per cent reduction in the risk of prostate cancer and a 36 per cent lowering of the risk of cancer spreading.

Those who consumed lots of tomatoes, but nevertheless developed prostate cancer, had a much less aggressive and life-threatening form of the disease. Indeed, in a paper published in 2007, Giovannucci concluded that the most significant role that tomatoes may play in prostate cancer could be that of slowing or stopping the non-aggressive form from progressing to become the aggressive form.

Summary

Dietary and lifestyle changes can play an important role in the growth of prostate cancer, although they do not replace drug therapy, surgery, chemotherapy or radiation therapy. Evidence is, however, accumulating that tomato and lycopene may not only reduce the risk of developing prostate cancer, but also enhance the effectiveness of current orthodox treatments and reduce the risk of the disease recurring. Moreover, there is evidence to suggest that the tomato's most important role could be to reduce, slow or prevent the conversion of latent prostate cancer to the aggressive lethal form.

Rudy Giuliani, former mayor of New York, 9/11 popular hero and 2008 US presidential candidate, declared some years ago that, since being diagnosed with prostate cancer, he has eaten large quantities of lycopene-rich tomatoes.

The evidence I have presented reflects the conclusions drawn by the vast majority of completed studies and reviews. It is, however, only right to point out that a small number of studies have failed to find a strong connection, or any at all, between tomato consumption and prostate cancer prevention. Even so, one of these – the very recently published EPIC study which involved 137,000 men in eight European countries – found that while evidence of localised disease prevention was lacking, there was strong evidence that the risk of developing advanced, and therefore more dangerous, disease was considerably reduced in men with the highest blood lycopene levels.

Such is the nature of things in the biological, especially medical, sciences!

Postscript

In November 2007, the most comprehensive, independent and expert analysis yet of the link between our food choices and our susceptibility to all cancers was published by the World Cancer

Research Fund and the American Institute for Cancer Research. Entitled *Food, Nutrition, Physical Activity, and the Prevention of Cancer*, it required more than 100 leading international medical and nutrition scientists to scrutinise over 7,000 published studies over a period of some three years.

The following is an extract from the section devoted to prostate cancer:

'A total of 42 tomato/lycopene studies were reviewed ... those based on regular intake of lycopene, or of tomato sauce (from which lycopene is highly bioavailable*) showed a statistically significant decreased risk of developing prostate cancer ... Lycopene is best absorbed after the fruit (tomato) is cooked and puréed.

'The report emphasises that advanced and aggressive cancers may be better linked to prognosis[†] ... Lycopene is the most potent carotenoid antioxidant, has anti-proliferative effect, reduces blood LDL cholesterol, improves immune function and reduces inflammation.'

*easily absorbed
[†]may be most effective against more dangerous cancers

CHAPTER 6

Absorption, Safety and Mode of Action

In order for the health-protecting constituents of tomatoes to do their work, they must first be successfully absorbed into the body and distributed to the vulnerable tissues and organs which they can then help to safeguard. A number of factors influencing both absorption and distribution are discussed in this chapter.

Tomatoes are available in a wide variety of forms: raw, in cans, in sauce, sun-dried, powdered, puréed, juiced, in soups, in salsa, as pizza topping, in ketchup. All forms contain lycopene, but some have higher concentrations than others.

In 1995, Giovannucci and the Harvard Group published the results of a survey of 47,000 male health professionals who had been included in the

HPFS study. They found that tomato sauces and ketchups were far richer in lycopene than raw tomatoes and tomato juice. Evidently, the combination of cooking tomatoes and condensing them concentrated the lycopene that they contained. An examination of the Mediterranean diet also suggested that cooking tomatoes in the presence of olive oil did something to improve their potency.

It turned out that the valuable carotenoids – lycopene, beta-carotene, etc. – exist within a protein matrix. Heating tomatoes causes the matrix to break down, thereby releasing the carotenoids which are not soluble in water, but very soluble in oil. So cooking tomatoes in the presence of oil primes the carotenoids for absorption into the body.

According to an Italian study, absorption of lycopene is more than three times greater when consumed as tomato sauce, paste or tomato oleoresin capsules (see Chapter Eight) than from raw tomatoes. That study also found that a regular daily intake of tomatoes, equivalent to 6–8 mg of lycopene, was sufficient to increase resistance to cell DNA oxidation damage, and that regular intake of small quantities of tomato is essential to maintaining protective levels.

Absorption is improved when the cooking or heat processing is carried out in the presence of a suitable edible oil, e.g. olive oil, sunflower oil and rapeseed oil. For example, an Australian study compared blood lycopene concentration following consumption of diced tomatoes cooked (a) with a little extra virgin olive oil, and (b) without any oil. The former was found to produce considerably higher blood levels of lycopene.

The important part played by fats in the absorption of lycopene is well illustrated by the fact that when synthetic fats, i.e. fat substitutes such as sucrose polyesters, are consumed within the diet, they dissolve some of the lycopenee. However, as they themselves are not absorbed, they carry the antioxidant through the gut to be excreted, and 30 per cent of the lycopene is lost.

Other factors that can affect the amount of lycopene reaching the bloodstream include the composition of the diet in general. For example, high-fibre diets can absorb lycopene molecules. As with synthetic fats, a loss of lycopene can occur.

Stability

Lycopene is stable both in the raw fruit matrix and when freed by heating. However, when isolated in its pure form, it is vulnerable to degradation by light and oxygen. It is therefore stored by manufacturers and processors under nitrogen and in darkness: an inert environment.

How does the absorption of lycopene and other carotenoids take place?

The absorption process begins in the stomach, where the carotenoid-bearing oil droplets are subjected to normal digestive processes, leading to the small intestine where they pass through the intestinal lining and into the bloodstream. Lycopene makes its way to the liver, the main storage site, from where it is transported, as part of a lipoprotein (LDL) complex, to the tissues.

Once absorbed, carotenoids are not uniformly distributed in the body, but become concentrated in certain areas. This is thought to be influenced by the fact that specific carotenoids can exert unique biological effects in certain tissues but not in others. For example, the two carotenoids lutein and zeaxanthin make their way almost exclusively to the macula, a tiny spot within the retina through which light must pass to form an image. It is believed that they quench damaging free radicals and absorb excessive and blue light, thereby protecting the retina from possible damage by oxidation. This may be the origin of the old adage that carrots help one see in the dark.

Other than the liver, the highest amounts of lycopene are to be found in the blood, lungs, adrenal glands, testes and prostate, while lower concentrations are present in the pancreas, colon, kidneys, breast, skin, breast milk, cervix, ovaries and spleen.

Safety of tomato and lycopene

According to Paula Trumbo at the FDA Centre for Safety and Applied Nutrition, lycopene did not show any significant adverse effect in acute medium or long-term safety studies. In pregnancy there was no evidence that lycopene is toxic to either the mother or the foetus. She concluded that 'the data suggests there were no observed adverse effects at a dose level as high as the equivalent of 3 g per kg/day', i.e. 100 to 1,000 times the recommended adult intake.

Everson and McQueen also reviewed the safety of lycopene and noted that no adverse lycopene effects, precautions or contraindications had been reported. They concluded that 'lycopene, or a diet high in lycopene, can safely be recommended for prostate cancer prevention or as supportive therapy'. Writing in the *Sight and Life Newsletter*, McClaren wrote: 'No evidence has ever been found of toxicity from high consumption of lycopene.'

Lycopene appears to possess an inbuilt safety mechanism. Following absorption, irrespective of the dose or the period of consumption, lycopene blood levels never rise beyond a level which is both safe and fortunately also very effective. In an absorption trial, doses as high as 75 mg per day did not even reach that safe level. Absorbed lycopene that is surplus to the body's requirements is apparently excreted unchanged.

Tomatoes and acidity

For many years the tomato was regarded as an acid-forming food which would increase the acidity of the blood and body tissues. Because of this, sufferers of gout and arthritis were advised not to eat tomatoes. The latest studies in nutritional chemistry have completely dispelled these ideas as baseless. Indeed, the tomato is now considered beneficial in the treatment of acidosis and other diseases associated with excessive acidity in the system.

How could tomato and lycopene work against cancer?

In the year 2000, the scientists responsible for producing the *White Book* concluded that 'oxidative DNA damage gives rise to DNA mutations and is therefore implicated in cancer initiation'.

Previously, and with some foresight, in a comprehensive review published in 1981, the Oxford group Peto, Doll, Buckley and Sporn wrote:

'There is growing evidence that retinoids and perhaps carotenoids may be anti-cancer agents ... possible mechanisms include protection by carotenoids of target tissues by enhancing some immune function or by quenching singlet oxygen, a highly reactive excited molecule generated during normal metabolic processes ... it seems probable a few truly protective agents do await discovery among a dozen or so dietary factors of current interest.'

The singlet oxygen radical, mentioned above, is a very reactive high-energy oxygen fragment that is produced during everyday metabolism. It can attack and damage DNA and blood fats. Lycopene could intervene to neutralise the radical, thereby rendering it harmless.

Sian Astley, at the Institute of Food Research in Norwich, reported having found more than 60 published *in vivo* studies that showed a DNA-related response to lycopene. She concluded that an increase in the lycopene concentration in the blood or in the target cells, e.g. in the prostate, 'is consistently associated with decreased DNA damage or increased repair in target tissue'.

Phyllis Bowen's team at the University of Illinois have been studying the effect of lycopene on cancer development for many years, and have found several possible ways in which lycopene could act against cancer. For example, it decreases the blood concentration of those hormones known to stimulate prostate cancer growth (IGF-1), and also has anti-inflammatory properties.

Lycopene's outstanding ability to block the DNA-damaging potential of singlet oxygen, and other unwelcome free radicals, led initially to the assumption that this explains lycopene's apparent anti-cancer activity. However, several animal, human and tissue/cell laboratory studies have shown that lycopene benefits health in a surprising number of additional ways, which are probably interdependent, and include the following:

1. IGF-1 suppression

IGF-1 is an insulin-like growth factor manufactured in the liver, which is known to stimulate the growth and spread of prostate and breast cancer. Three independent studies have each concluded that lycopene may suppress excessive production of IGF-1.

In a study with prostate cancer patients awaiting surgery, the oncologist Kucuk found that, when compared to untreated control patients, those who received lycopene supplementation showed a 29 per cent reduction in IGF-1 blood levels.

An editorial that appeared in the *British Medical Journal* in 2000 agreed that high levels of IGF-1 may increase the possibility of body cells becoming cancerous, or may obstruct an important part of the body's own anti-cancer defences.

2. Inter-cellular communication

Another possible mechanism is based on evidence that lycopene enhances what is called 'gap junctional communication' between cells. Gap junctions are water-filled pores that connect neighbouring cells, thereby enabling chemical communication between cells. This process plays a role in the regulation of all differentiation in cell growth and apoptosis, or the death of tumour cells. It has been speculated that such increased contact between cells may even reverse the malignant process.

3. Cholesterol reduction

High blood cholesterol levels are believed to accelerate, but not initiate, prostate cancer growth by helping the tumours to withstand anti-cancer defences. In a laboratory study, lycopene was found to inhibit the activity of a particular enzyme which is essential for cholesterol synthesis. A small clinical study has provided evidence suggesting that lycopene may indeed have a cholesterol-lowering effect, similar to that produced by taking statin medication, but without the same risk of side effects.

A number of other possible explanations for the beneficial effects of tomato constituents are being investigated, but meanwhile they all remain hypotheses that are supported by evidence, but still awaiting definitive testing.

Conclusion

'Lycopene acts via different mechanisms that have potential to co-operatively delay cell cycle progression in prostate epithelial cells, to reduce DNA damage and improve oxidative stress defence.'

Taken from the Executive Summary page of the *White Book*

According to a recently published review by Keith Block of the University of Illinois, contrary to previous assumptions, when patients on chemotherapy are given antioxidants such as those present in tomatoes, the effect is to improve survival rates, tumour response and patients' ability to tolerate the chemotherapy.

CHAPTER 7

The Tomato Versus Other Serious Conditions

It is widely believed that a whole array of diseases, ailments, illnesses, conditions, disorders – call them what you will – are associated with free radical damage. Naturally this means that age enters the equation too, making older people more likely to become unwell.

Investigations into the protective role tomatoes might play have therefore been initiated in a wide variety of complaints. None of the evidence can, at present, be said to be more than interesting, but it is not discouraging either. Much more research will be necessary before definite conclusions can be drawn. Meanwhile, to provide the reader with a sense of what the future may hold:

Pre-eclampsia

This is a life-threatening condition that arises in pregnancy. It is characterised by high blood pressure, fluid retention and proteinuria (protein in the urine). A test group of 251 pregnant women was divided in two. One group received 2 mg of lycopene daily, while the other group received a placebo. During the course of gestation 8.6 per cent of the first group developed pre-eclampsia, while 17.7 per cent of the second group did so. Delayed growth in the uterus, an early sign of pre-eclampsia, occurred in 12 per cent of the lycopene group and 23.7 per cent of the control placebo group. The authors concluded that, while lycopene supplementation appeared to be beneficial, confirmation in much larger numbers of women must be awaited.

A recently published critical review of seven published studies involving over 6,000 women concluded that, while the quality of the studies was variable and conclusions were drawn with caution, nevertheless antioxidant supplements, and not only tomatoes, seemed to reduce the risk of pre-eclampsia.

Eye diseases

Age-related Macular Degeneration (AMD) affects the tiny central part of the retina called the macula which controls fine vision, leaving sufferers with only limited sight at best. It affects more than 30 million people worldwide.

Researchers Mares and Moeller reviewed a large number of published investigations to check whether or not diet is associated with the development of AMD, a leading cause of blindness in the Western world and one for which there is no satisfactory treatment. They found that where diets were higher in antioxidants (vitamins C and E, carotenoids, fruits, vegetables and zinc) the eye disease was less frequent and less severe.

This serious eye condition is thought to start with damage to eye tissue caused by excessive exposure to bright sunlight. Ultraviolet and blue light cause the release, within the eye, of free radicals, which attack molecules in the eye tissue leading to oxidation and inflammation. As they age, eyes lose their natural antioxidant defence. The two researchers found 'a substantial body of evidence which supports the proposition that several dietary constituents have a role in protecting sensitive eye tissues'.

Another group of scientists, who had also studied the role of antioxidants in the prevention of eye disease, concluded that a mixture of antioxidants is more effective than high doses of a single one – a theme which has been cropping up with increasing frequency. Realising that dealing with well-developed AMD is difficult and far from satisfactory, these authors suggested that the most successful way to avoid oxidative eye diseases is to adopt healthy dietary practices at an early stage.

In the eye, the macula is the region of greatest visual acuity. It sits near the centre of the retina at the back of the eyeball. In 1997 scientists discovered that the yellow colour of the macula was due to the presence of two carotenoids, lutein and zeaxanthin. It has been suggested that they protect the retina from light damage by absorbing excess ultraviolet and blue light. They may also quench free radicals generated by sunlight exposure. This research group subsequently went on to identify a diverse mixture of carotenoids in various eye tissues, including the iris and lens, where they believe the carotenoids can help prevent or delay cataract formation.

The results of a major clinical trial called AREDS, involving 4,500 participants aged 60–80 and supported by the US National Eye Institute, was published in September 2007. It added further scientific weight to earlier findings that high dietary intakes of carotenoids, especially lutein and zeaxanthin, can decrease risk of developing AMD very significantly.

Osteoporosis

In this condition, bones become fragile and brittle due to loss of elasticity and reduction in bone mass. Although the number of published studies is small, one study being undertaken, by Leticia Rao and colleagues at St Michael's Hospital, Toronto, warrants a special mention. According to Rao, osteoporosis is a major metabolic disease suffered by one in four women over the age of 50 and by a significant proportion of men too. In women, it is prompted by the reduction in oestrogen levels when they reach menopause.

Bone is not a permanent tissue. On the contrary, it is constantly renewing itself through a process involving removal of old bone and formation of new bone. According to Rao, it is widely accepted that oxidative stress is responsible for an imbalance that occurs, leading to bone loss outpacing the formation of new bone. From their preliminary studies the Toronto team concluded that lycopene, acting as an antioxidant, appeared to reduce both oxidative stress and signs of excessive bone turnover. From this, they hoped that dietary lycopene might have an important role to play in reducing the risk of osteoporosis.

Their hypothesis is being put to the test in a major study. The final results are expected to show whether dietary lycopene can be used alone as a treatment for osteoporosis, or as a complement to standard drug treatments.

Male infertility

According to male infertility specialist Armand Zini, infertility affects 15 per cent of couples and in 30–50 per cent of these cases the problem is with the male. Human sperm is particularly vulnerable to oxidative damage, due to the abundance of unsaturated fatty acids in the sperm membrane. Excess production, or inadequate on-the-spot control, of free radicals released in the semen leads to sperm cell damage. High levels of free radicals have been found to be present in 25–40 per cent of infertile men. The effect of oxidative stress on semen is to reduce sperm numbers and cause low motility. Lycopene is a normal constituent of the testes and semen, where its presence seems essential.

In 1996, a study carried out with infertile men was published. In it the investigators had given 2 mg of lycopene, twice daily for three months, to men with extremely low sperm counts. Their results showed improvements in both sperm motility and numbers.

Preliminary studies have shown that infertile men often have lower semen lycopene concentrations than fertile men. A research group undertook a study to check the usefulness of lycopene in the treatment of 50 patients with no obvious cause for their infertility. Each patient was given a lycopene oleoresin capsule (see Chapter Eight), containing 8 mg of lycopene, daily until their sperm analysis was normalised or pregnancy was achieved. Results showed a 36 per cent pregnancy success rate.

Skin cancer

Skin cancer rates in Britain have doubled in the past twenty years. The principal cause is excessive sunlight exposure, which causes more free radicals to be released within the skin. They damage skin fat, protein and DNA resulting in premature skin ageing, light-sensitisation and skin cancers.

To check whether lycopene could influence this damage, nine volunteers were given tomato paste together with olive oil, daily, for ten weeks. At the end of this time patches of their skin were exposed to levels of artificial sunlight sufficient to cause erythema (sunburn and inflammation). Those who had taken tomato paste suffered 40 per cent less erythema than those who consumed only olive oil. The researchers concluded that it might be possible to protect skin against erythema simply by consuming adequate quantities of lycopene-rich foods, i.e. lots of tomatoes.

In another study, 25 volunteers took an anti-oxidant mixture (lycopene, beta-carotene, vitamin E and selenium) daily for seven weeks. The researchers noted a number of improvements in the skin's defences against UV-induced damage, and concluded that the mixture could provide a 'safe, daylong and efficient complement to sun-screen skin applications and may help reduce DNA damage, skin ageing and skin cancer'.

Additional positive evidence came from yet another study. This time volunteers were given one of three alternative forms of lycopene, each equivalent to 10 mg a day for twelve weeks. When then exposed to artificial sunlight designed to produce erythema, synthetic lycopene alone reduced the severity of erythema by 25 per cent, whereas the natural tomato-derived versions led to reductions of 38 per cent and 48 per cent. This led the investigators to conclude that the extra carotenoids present in whole tomatoes had enhanced the action of the lycopene.

Lycopene has also been incorporated into a skin cream. Its performance against artificial sunlight exposure was then compared with that of a cream containing vitamins C and E. The results showed that the lycopene cream provided much greater protection from skin damage.

Many studies have shown that when the concentrations of certain carotenoids (lycopene, lutein and zeaxanthin) are raised in the skin through increased consumption, they can help protect the skin from UV-induced damage. This very important finding has prompted the manufacturers of beauty and skincare products to introduce a new concept in protection. That is, protecting not only the skin surface, but also the much more vulnerable deeper layers, by means of capsules containing lycopene and other carotenoids. A study published in 2007 showed that a combination of these, taken both internally and applied to the skin, increases protection sixfold. In addition, the combined approach led to improved skin appearance by increasing elasticity, hydration and surface skin fat.

According to a report in the *Daily Mail* on 10

July 2007, sunscreen manufacturers have agreed to stop using terms such as 'total sun block', '100 per cent protection' or 'total protection', as skin cancer experts have declared that no product can protect the skin entirely. Ultraviolet-A is the type of sunlight associated with skin cancer. According to the cancer charity RAFT (Restoration of Appearance and Function Trust), most creams provide no protection against ultraviolet-A when rubbed into the skin, rather than left on the surface as a film.

From the research, it would appear that there is a case for increasing one's lycopene consumption, as well as applying a good sunscreen, to provide better protection before significant sun exposure.

Gastric cancer

In 1994 Italian researchers reported a survey which showed a protective effect from lycopene in a wide variety of digestive tract cancers among people who habitually ate seven or more helpings of tomatoes each week. A reduction in the risk of upper respiratory and digestive tract cancer, from daily tomato consumption, was also reported in two other surveys.

Dr Yuan and colleagues at the Norris Cancer Centre in Los Angeles had access to the dietary records of a major study carried out in Shanghai, involving volunteers who had been monitored over a period of twelve years. Their blood concentrations of beta-carotene and lycopene had been measured at the outset of the study. After twelve years, 191 of the volunteers had developed gastric cancer. Their original blood data were compared with those of 570 matched cancer-free control volunteers. The investigators found that those individuals with the highest levels of the carotenoids, especially lycopene, at the outset showed the lowest risk of developing the disease.

Another ten-year study involved 3,182 subjects drawn from rural Japan. This also showed that those who had started out with the highest lycopene blood levels had the lowest risk.

It is still very early days, and much more work needs to be done before reliable conclusions can be drawn.

Lung cancer

According to Greg Whyte, former Olympic athlete and now Professor of Sport and Exercise Science and Physiology at Liverpool John Moores University, pollution of the environment is mainly due to emissions from road vehicles. Ozone is produced when sunlight reacts with combustion gases, giving rise to highly reactive free radicals which inflame the lining of the lungs.

Because lungs are constantly exposed to the environment – dust, smoke and pathogens – they have an extensive defence system, in which lycopene already plays a part.

In a study of 103 Spanish women who had been diagnosed with lung cancer, their normal tomato consumption was recorded and compared with that of 206 matched controls who were free of lung disease. This study showed that the higher the regular consumption of tomatoes had been, the lower the apparent risk of developing lung cancer.

A much longer study was carried out in southwest England, when the consumption of fifteen dietary constituents was monitored for a period of four years. At the end of this time, the initial total food intakes of patients diagnosed with lung cancer was compared with those of matched healthy controls. The regular daily intake of as little as one medium-sized tomato appeared to have reduced the risk of lung cancer over the test period by some 30 per cent.

In Japan, 34,000 individuals took part in a major health study. Following blood measurements at the outset, dietary and illness records were gathered over a period of eight years. By referring to the initial recorded data, the investigators were able to conclude that the risk of developing lung cancer appeared lowest among individuals whose initial blood levels of lycopene and other carotenoids had been highest.

Type 2 diabetes

In the period immediately after eating, especially in diabetics, there are changes in blood chemistry which cause a sudden increase in the production of free radicals. This prompted some researchers to consider whether antioxidants, in particular lycopene, could have a role in the management of type 2 (adult onset) diabetes.

Using data gathered in the USA from 1998 to 1991 for the third National Health and Nutrition Survey, blood concentrations of several carotenoids were compared in individuals with (a) normal blood glucose tolerance, (b) abnormal blood glucose tolerance, and (c) newly diagnosed type 2 diabetes. Levels of both lycopene and beta-carotene were lowest where the condition was most advanced. The data suggested to the investigators the need for more research, seeking a possible beneficial role for carotenoids in reversing the development of type 2 diabetes.

Finnish researchers studied the relationship between blood carotenoid concentrations and the outcome of an oral blood glucose tolerance test in a group of some 200 individuals considered to be at high risk of developing type 2 diabetes. They concluded that the data suggests an advantageous association between carotenoids, especially beta-carotene, and glucose metabolism in men at high risk.

In Australia, some 1,600 volunteers had their blood concentrations of five carotenoids measured. They were then subjected to an oral glucose tolerance test. The authors noted that patients with the highest blood levels of carotenoids (alpha- and beta-carotene, betacryptoxanthin, lutein, zeaxanthin and lycopene), all of which are present in tomatoes, showed the smallest rise in blood glucose and lowest fasting insulin, both reflecting beneficial influences.

Asthma

According to Wood and colleagues at the John Hunter Hospital in New South Wales, Australia, elevated oxidative stress and impaired anti-oxidant defences are increasingly recognised phenomena in asthma research. They found that whole blood carotenoid levels were much lower in asthmatics than in non-asthmatic controls.

Asthma attacks can be induced by exercise. To check whether patients known to be sensitive to exercise could benefit from lycopene (i.e. anti-oxidant) supplementation, a small study was carried out in which twenty patients were given 30 mg of lycopene daily for a week. When subsequently exposed to risk of an exercise-induced asthma attack, 55 per cent were significantly protected against their usual symptoms. The authors concluded that a large, definitive trial was justified.

Inflammatory polyarthritis

Polyarthritis is an arthritic condition involving two or more joints. Researchers studied the dietary records of some 25,000 participants in the EPIC (European Prospective Investigation into Cancer and Nutrition) study. From these, they found that individuals who had regularly consumed a diet rich in the carotenoids zeaxanthin and betacryptoxanthin, both present in tomatoes, appeared to have reduced their risk of developing the disease. The association with betacryptoxanthin was said to be especially significant.

Venous thrombosis

This condition occurs when blood clots in the

veins, which can lead to sudden death. Blood platelet aggregation, or stickiness, plays an essential part in the formation of blood clots that can lead to venous thrombosis. A research group at the Rowett Institute in Aberdeen discovered, in the yellow jelly that surrounds tomato seeds, an extractive containing constituents that appear to inhibit platelet stickiness. This should thereby help to prevent, or at least impede, clot formation.

Ageing

According to a Greek adage, 'it is the function of medicine to help people die young as late as possible'. In 1956, Dr Denham Harman published his free radical explanation for ageing. In it he stated that all organisms, including humans, accumulate free radical damage to their proteins, fats and nucleic acids (i.e. DNA and RNA) over time. This damage leads to a reduction in their respective functions, thereby decreasing cell function, then organ function and, finally, all function.

The hypothesis is by no means universally accepted, but it does enjoy a fair amount of experimental support. In 1995 medical scientists at the Nutritional Research Center on Ageing at Tufts University in Boston published an important review of the relationship between antioxidants and immunity in older people. They concluded that, while low consumption of dietary antioxidants led to a decline in immune function, a higher intake resulted in better immune response.

While relatively little research has been conducted to date on the possible role of antioxidants in managing the ageing process, other than with the skin, that aspect will undoubtedly feature in future work. However, an example of their possible benefit was suggested by a recent French study of 589 highly educated, community-dwelling elderly men and women. Low blood levels of lycopene and zeaxanthin were found to be linked to poor cognitive function. The investigators concluded that natural cognitive decline with age might be slowed by consuming more of the relevant antioxidants.

From a symposium on healthy ageing held recently in Chicago came the important conclusion that antioxidants, calcium, vitamin D and zinc can slow the development of age-related diseases and increase a person's healthy life expectancy.

CHAPTER 8

From Farm to Pharmacy

The evidence to date shows that the most effective way of obtaining the health benefits of the tomato is to regularly consume whole fruits which have been cooked or heat processed in the presence of small quantities of olive oil. Results from studies in which the effectiveness of isolated pure lycopene was compared with that from equivalent amounts of whole fruits showed the latter to be more potent. This is taken to indicate that constituents present only in the whole fruits, albeit in minute concentrations, enhance the effectiveness of lycopene.

Scientists are testing to see whether the desiccation of tomatoes affects lycopene potency. If not, then it might be useful in administering doses to those who are reluctant to consume whole tomatoes, those who have difficulty in accessing fresh fruits and those who need a concentrated dosage.

The food, pharmaceutical and cosmetic industries have, since time immemorial, added substances designed to add colour in order to attract the consumer, creating and inspiring interest, desire and comfort. Natural pigments extracted from plants, flowers, minerals and even insects were the original sources but, being products of nature, they tend to vary in quality from batch to batch. They also require processing and offer a limited range of colours.

During the late 19th century and throughout the 20th, natural colouring agents were largely supplanted by synthetic chemicals, which offered an almost infinite choice of colours with reliable quality and stability. However, during the latter decades of the 20th century consumers became increasingly aware of, and concerned about, their possible long-term effects, and many of them are now banned for safety reasons. This led to a renewed interest in finding reliable, innocuous natural colouring agents.

One such agent is the carotenoid beta-carotene, which is normally present in human blood. It is not manufactured in the human body, but derived from our food. The main sources are carrots, spinach, sweet potato and pumpkin. Beta-carotene is a safe and very useful colourant at high dilution over the yellow–orange range. It is consumed by the majority of the world's population every day in foods, medicines, cosmetics and other products.

Nutritional studies carried out in the 1960s and 1970s appeared to show that many major chronic diseases, such as cancers and heart diseases, might be initiated by a common factor: exposure to free radicals released in the body in the course of normal metabolism. Following the discovery that beta-carotene was a powerful antioxidant, the suggestion arose that perhaps, if it were present in the tissues in adequate concentration, it might render the free radicals harmless as quickly as they were generated.

Accordingly, clinical studies were initiated. Demand for natural beta-carotene, to be used in much higher concentration as an ingredient in dietary supplements, soon followed. A rich source is the pink alga *Dunaliella salina*. It can be grown quickly and easily, and an Israeli company named Koor Foods soon developed a commercially successful method of growing the alga in order to extract the carotenoid.

In 1989, a study was published which was the first to report that lycopene possessed even more powerful antioxidant properties. This led scientists to investigate whether lycopene had anything to offer in the fight against cancer and other major chronic diseases. From the previous chapters you, the reader, will know the answer.

Koor scientists, led by Dov Hartel, undertook an urgent study to find a means of producing natural lycopene in commercial quantities. Lycopene is present in watermelons, apricots, pink grapefruit and several exotic fruits, but is found in much higher quantities in tomatoes.

Tomatoes are grown in bulk and processed into soups, juices, pasta sauces, etc. in several countries, including Israel. The process gives rise to large quantities of tomato waste in the form of skin and seeds, to which the Koor team turned initially. The extraction of lycopene from this was successful but uneconomic. Lycopene is plentiful in the pulp which, being the greater bulk, was more likely to provide a plentiful supply. Even so, the lycopene content was very small: about 50 mg per kg. But what, they wondered, if tomatoes can be induced to increase their lycopene content?

Hartel turned to the late Professor Raphael Frenkel, a leading international authority on tomato breeding, for advice. Using only traditional breeding methods and without resorting to genetic manipulation, Frenkel and Hartel soon developed a tomato variety that tripled typical lycopene content. This variety is known as LRT, or lycopene-rich tomato. By 1991, Koor had built a plant for processing the tomatoes. A new company was launched with the specific aim of producing, in a commercially viable way, high-quality tomato lycopene for use both as a harmless food colourant and, in much higher concentration, as a dietary supplement.

The new company, LycoRed Natural Product Industries Ltd, had shown great foresight and initiative since, within the decade, the health role of tomatoes and the demand for a reliable whole tomato concentrated extract would arise. In 1992 LycoRed became a subsidiary of Makhteshim Agan Industries Ltd, a leading agricultural chemicals company and one of Israel's largest industrial groups.

The production process

According to LycoRed, LRT plants are cultivated under careful control with minimal use of agrochemicals. Harvested when red ripe, the tomatoes are then transported to the processing plant, where they are sorted and washed to remove residual agrochemicals. As tomatoes are a seasonal product, the processing operation is carried out in two stages. First the pulp is prepared from the ripe fruit and kept frozen at a temperature of minus 18 °C (or minus 0.4 °F) under vacuum. The pulp can then be used throughout the ensuing year to produce the final product. Each batch is tracked so that, if necessary, it can be traced back to a particular lot in the field.

The extraction method used by LycoRed is subject to US Patent number 5837311. After washing and sorting, the tomatoes are crushed and spun at high speed to separate the pulp from the juice. The pulp is analysed, to ensure that it contains at least 500 ppm (parts per million) lycopene, before being finely ground and frozen.

When required, frozen pulp is transferred to the extraction plant, where it is mixed and agitated with solvents in which lycopene and other fat-soluble nutrients are dissolved. The mixture is then filtered, and the nutrient containing the filtrate evaporated under vacuum, to ensure the removal of solvents. This leaves a concentrated extract containing lycopene and other tomato nutrients dissolved in the natural tomato oils, among them oleic and linoleic oils. The extract, which is known as tomato oleoresin, is then blended with other tomato oleoresin batches to produce standard, reproducible oleoresin. The oleoresin is essentially whole tomato, minus its 95 per cent water content.

According to LycoRed, the ratio between lycopene and other oil-soluble constituents in oleoresin closely reflects that present in the original tomatoes (see Table 1 on the next page). The standard oleoresin, which is marketed worldwide as 'Lyc-O-Mato', is provided in a variety of physical forms for incorporation into liquid and solid food and cosmetic products. The pure oleoresin is used in dietary supplement capsules, in which form it has participated in numerous published and ongoing clinical studies. The specification for Lyc-O-Mato 15 mg soft gel capsules is shown in Table 2. LycoRed claims that each capsule provides the lycopene and other carotenoid content of six large ripe tomatoes.

To check that the oleoresin form would be adequately absorbed and distributed within the body, a study was carried out with 75 patients due to undergo haemorrhoid removal. Capsules of oleoresin (30 mg/day) or placebo were given for one to seven weeks prior to surgery. The surgically removed tissues were subsequently examined for lycopene content. Blood, skin and fatty tissue concentrations were found to have doubled in the treated patients compared to the control individuals, thereby confirming satisfactory absorption.

Table 1: Comparison of active ingredient ratios in tomato and Lyc-O-Mato

(data supplied by LycoRed)

	Ratio to total lycopene in ripe tomato	Ratio to total lycopene in Lyc-O-Mato
Lycopene	100.0	100.0
Phytoene	10.0	10.0
Phytofluene	9.1	9.0
Vitamin E	34.5	33.3

Table 2: Composition of tomato oleoresin – mg of active ingredients

Lycopene	15.0
Phytoene	1.5
Phytofluene	1.25
Tocopherols	5.0
Phytosterols	1.5

When foods were first identified as possessing health-promoting quasi-medicinal properties, the assumption was made that within those foods could be found individual constituents which were responsible for those beneficial properties. These would be identified, extracted, purified and concentrated, or even synthesised, with a view to incorporating them into tablets or capsules. The carotenoid beta-carotene was one such example.

Clinical trials were run, in the expectation of obtaining results similar to those obtained with foods rich in beta-carotene. However, nutritional and medical scientists were puzzled when the expected results were not forthcoming. Their first instincts were to assume that the construction of the trial might have been wrong. Dosage too high or too low? Incorrect patient selection? Too short a trial period? Too few patients for reliable statistical assessment?

The beta-carotene experience was almost repeated with lycopene, but this time it quickly became clear that results obtained with lycopene were not equalled when pure lycopene, whether natural or synthetic, was used. The conclusion was that lycopene comes complete with minute quantities of other tomato constituents that enhance, sometimes quite dramatically, the action of lycopene alone. Nature's ways are neither simple nor direct, one might say.

LycoRed scientists appear to have recognised

this distinction early on, and therefore set about producing a concentrate which would reproduce the total effects of the original fruit. Versions of the oleoresin that are suitable for incorporation into foods and beverages such as pasta, baked products, drinks, yoghurt, smoothies and cereals have been marketed worldwide by LycoRed. The products received approval from the UK Food Standards Agency for incorporation at a level up to 5 mg of lycopene per serving, an amount that is claimed to be sufficient to provide health benefits.

CHAPTER 9

On the Record

This chapter comprises ten quotations, each taken directly from the original publications of independent international nutritional researchers. References to the publication sources are provided.

'That nutrition was so largely ignored in practise may have been partly because of reluctance to consider anything so banal as that which we eat could contribute to the production of cancer.'

Richard Doll, *Nutrition and Cancer*,
Vol. 1, pp. 35–45, 1978

'There is growing evidence that retinoids and perhaps carotenoids may be anti-carcinogenic.'

Peto, Doll, Buckley and Sporn, *Nature*,
Vol. 290, p. 201–08, 1981

'It is clear that tomatoes have a significant contribution to make in terms of public health, thanks to their antioxidant content ... Many diseases involve oxidation processes, i.e. free radicals, in their evolution. Antioxidants lycopene, vitamins C and E are able to capture free radicals, reducing disease induction ... the protective role of antioxidant-rich diets in disease protection and ageing are beyond doubt.'

White Book, 2000, extract from 'Conclusions'

'... it is evident from published studies we have reviewed that the incidence of prostate and lung cancer can be lowered by adequate intake of tomato products.'

G. Muller et al, *Current Opinion in Clinical Nutrition Metabolism*, Vol. 6, pp. 657–60, 2003

'Lycopene is bound to the skin and fibre in fresh tomatoes and is less available [for absorption] in uncooked than cooked tomatoes. Mild cooking disrupts the cell structure of the tomato, making it more available.

This report suggests that lycopene or lycopene in conjunction with other substances present in tomatoes may be a viable bioactive compound in the prevention of some cancer.'

E. Hwang and P. Bowen, *Integrative Cancer Therapies*, Vol. 1, pp. 121–32, 2002

'... overall, data suggest that the intake of tomato and tomato products is associated with decreased risk of prostate cancer.'

E. Giovannucci, *Journal of the National Cancer Institute*, Vol. 94, pp. 391–8, 2002

'... if you are trying to reduce the risk of CHD or prostate cancer a diet that regularly contains tomatoes appears to be a healthy and beneficial choice.'

K. Cannene-Adams et al, *Journal of Nutrition*, Vol. 135, pp. 1226–30, 2005

'... lycopene acts via different mechanisms that have potential ... to reduce DNA damage and to improve oxidative stress defence. These provide plausible explanations for the epidemiological findings that lycopene can contribute to reduce prostate cancer risk.'

K. Wertz et al, *Archives Biochemistry and Biophysics*, Vol. 430, pp. 12–34, 2004

'Evidence is extensive enough to support increased consumption of tomato products, especially processed products, from which lycopene is most readily available.'

M. Fraser et al, *Expert Review of Anticancer Therapy*, Vol. 5, pp. 847–54, 2005

'Lycopene has emerged as a unique choice in the chemoprevention and treatment of various cancers. More convincing results in recent clinical trials are opening new avenues for treatment of advanced or refractory prostate cancer where maintenance of the quality of life is the primary end point.'

P. Bowen, *Biochimica et Biophysica Acta*, Vol. 1740, pp. 202–05, 2005

'... consumption of processed tomato products, including tomato oleoresin, is of significant health benefit, attributable to the combination of naturally occurring nutrients in tomatoes.'

A. Basu and V. Imrhan, *European Journal of Clinical Nutrition*, Vol. 61, pp. 295–303, 2007

CHAPTER 10

The Quality is in the Breeding

There is a perception among consumers that the tomatoes currently on sale do not enjoy the sweet fine flavour and aroma of those which are home grown or which we remember buying in the past. This apparent change may stem from modern breeding and growing methods. These methods are designed to produce tomatoes that are resistant to pests and disease, that have greater shelf life and that are capable of being packed and transported over long distances (often 1,000 miles and more) from the farm to the retailer, without deterioration.

Another explanation may lie in current hydroponic production practices, by which the tomato plants are grown not in soil but with their roots immersed in carefully formulated, nutrient-rich mineral water solutions. These are placed in very long troughs located in vast glasshouses, and the atmosphere in which the plants are grown is computer-controlled for temperature and humidity.

Commercial growers are aware of consumer concerns, and have encouraged horticultural scientists to explore ways and means of producing ripe fruits that are, and remain, sweet, tasty and firm while retaining the physical robustness already described. This has proved difficult to achieve. Because each and every change in breeding and growing conditions takes several seasons to assess, it is necessarily a slow process.

One obvious method, which has not yet been met with favour by the tomato-consuming public, is genetic modification. This could provide breeders with far more scope to meet the desired specifications. In 2002, researchers at the Purdue University in Indiana and the US Department of Agriculture Research Service announced that, using genetic technology, they had produced tomatoes with improved qualities. These are presently still at the research stage. Commercial production is not expected before 2010 and may never happen.

In an effort to assuage critical public opinion in the USA that growing GM tomatoes might 'contaminate' other crops, the US Department of

Agriculture's Biotechnology Regulating Service issued a statement drawing attention to the following facts:

1. Tomato plants are self-pollinating and naturally inbreed; the life of exposed pollen is short.
2. Tomatoes do not cross-pollinate with other plants; there is no evidence that GM tomatoes can cross-pollinate non-GM tomato plants in the vicinity.
3. No mechanism is known to exist in nature that would allow genetic material from a GM tomato plant to be transferred to anything other than another GM tomato plant.

There are more traditional methods of influencing the quality of the fruits. These include cross-breeding existing varieties to produce even more varieties, modifying each and every aspect of the growing conditions (temperature, light, moisture and exposure to sunlight, too much of which can be destructive), and changing the composition of the plants' own food sources.

Consumers are aware that there is a difference in aroma and flavour between ripe, partially ripe and unripe tomatoes. Horticultural scientists are also interested in the underlying factors that can influence the qualities of the fruit, such as firmness and resistance to pests and diseases. Today's horticulturalists are, moreover, required to help growers meet new, additional specifications, namely increasing the content of constituents that provide health benefits to consumers.

Studies carried out at tomato research stations include checking the effect of changing environmental conditions on antioxidant tomato components and their activity. These conditions can affect the antioxidant (i.e. beneficial) content quite significantly. Below are examples of the environmental tests that have been carried out at such facilities.

1. Greenhouse tomatoes, harvested at six different times of the year, were compared for their antioxidant content. Greenhouse cultivation produced higher levels of lycopene through most of the year, except for midsummer when temperatures exceed 30 °C (86 °F).

2. Comparing the effect of growing in different nutrient mineral solutions, chicken manure and grass clover caused no difference in yields, but the acidity of the fruit, vitamin C and lycopene content were all influenced by the nutritional source.

3. When ripe tomatoes were stored for ten days at 7 °C (44.5 °F), 15 °C (59 °F) and 25 °C

(77 °F), the lycopene content at the latter two temperatures was found to have increased twofold compared with those stored at 7 °C.

It is now known that lycopene production in commercially grown tomatoes takes place at 12–32 °C (53.5–89.5 °F), with the most favourable range being 22–25 °C (71.5–77 °F) in the presence of sunlight.

As previously mentioned Israeli horticulturalists, using traditional methods only, have developed a variety of tomato that produces a threefold increase in the content of lycopene and other carotenoids. Since it was developed specifically for use in forms from which the pro-health constituents can be extracted, issues of flavour and longevity did not arise.

A purple super-bodyguard

People who frequently consume red wines, blueberries and red grapes have been found to suffer some major chronic diseases less frequently than those who do not. Nutritional researchers have identified a family of antioxidant pigments, somewhat parallel to carotenoids, as the constituents that benefit health. These are known chemically as anthocyanins. In recent years numerous studies have shown that anthocyanins exert a wide range of biological effects which could help prevent or reduce serious chronic illnesses.

Researchers at Oregon State University recalled that among the wild varieties of tomato still growing in the Andes, there was one which was purple in colour. Examination of samples revealed that the colour was due to anthocyanins, and that these were being produced by a gene that is naturally present in this unique tomato variety.

Insofar as anthocyanins appear to possess health-promoting properties, one of the researchers, a graduate student, had a hunch that if that wild variety could be crossed with a popular commercial variety, it might produce a tomato that offers the benefits of combined pro-health constituents. That combination could turn out to be more potent than either parent plant.

The result of subsequent experimental work, based on traditional methods, was the production of a domestic type of tomato containing the purple pigment. The opportunity had been created for developing anthocyanin-rich tomatoes with enhanced health-promoting properties. The qualities and properties of the purple fruit, the skin of which is as dark as the aubergine, are currently being assessed. The scientists involved in this remarkable achievement estimate that purple tomatoes could hit salad plates soon after 2010.

Organic versus non-organic

Among the tomato-buying public there are many who believe that organically grown produce is superior to that grown by current commercial methods. To check this claim, experiments were conducted by researchers at Fort Pierce, a horticultural research station in Florida. Tomatoes grown by standard methods were compared for quality with fruit grown organically. No differences could be detected in their colour, firmness or acidity, but members of a taste panel were able to identify the organic produce by flavour, aroma and texture. Panellists preferred the organic product. The research team concluded that organic production may affect eating qualities, but that more taste testing was required before definite conclusions could be drawn.

In the belief that organic farming might produce a higher nutrient content, a study was carried out by the World Vegetable Centre in Taiwan. Organic and conventional soil systems were compared for the ripe fruit content of beta-carotene, lycopene, vitamin C and antioxidant activity. No differences could be detected other than that the organic fruit was less acidic, which may imply higher sugar content. However, Professor Alyson Mitchell and colleagues at the University of California carried out a ten-year study, which found that the organic tomatoes produced a much higher content of two flavonoid antioxidants that had previously been noted for a possible role in the prevention of heart disease.

The taste and flavour of tomatoes are influenced by several factors: sugars for sweetness, acids for tartness, the sugar/acid ratio, volatile compounds for aroma and the texture of the flesh. All of these factors interact when tasting, which is in itself very subjective. A good taste will have the right combination of sugars, acids, aroma and texture.

CHAPTER 11

A Tomato a Day ...

In 1954, scientists working at the Medical Research Council in London published a groundbreaking study. It confirmed earlier suspicions of a direct association between smoking and lung cancer. The paper was treated with derision because it was based on epidemiological (i.e. population) studies, which were not deemed seriously scientific at the time. Such studies are carried out by questioning and monitoring several thousand volunteers about aspects of their lifestyle over very extensive periods, five to twelve years or more, some being questioned over a period of half a century.

Within a decade of the appearance of the 1954 paper, its conclusions had been quite widely accepted by the medical profession, and today one would be hard pressed to find any serious dissenters. That publication by Richard Doll and Bradford Hill established, beyond doubt, the potential validity of epidemiological studies.

The evidence for the role of tomato lycopene that is presented in this book was initiated by a series of epidemiological studies which, together, have monitored over 200,000 individuals over periods of up to twelve years. The first significant epidemiological study that found a beneficial association between prostate cancer and tomato consumption appeared in 1995. It too was, and still is, treated with disbelief, especially by the medical establishment who say that it will require a safety and efficacy assessment similar to that required for a pharmaceutical medication to convince them.

However, one very influential medical scientist, specialising in the prevention of prostate cancer research, who was originally very sceptical, recently wrote an article reversing his former scepticism. This was published in February 2007 in *PCRI Insights*, the bulletin of the US Prostate Cancer Research Institute. Addressing its medical readers, Jacek Pinski MD, Professor of Medicine at the University of Southern California stated:

'It was considered medical heresy to suggest dietary supplements might play a constructive role in the battle against prostate cancer. Fortunately a bold community of scientific researchers ignored that ethic. Thanks to their efforts we now have a body of solid evidence on which to stand when we claim that natural ingredients can prolong prostate vitality ... and prevent prostate cancer cells from developing ... and may even prompt cancer cell death in men who have the disease. I am not suggesting natural supplements replace established treatments. They can play an important role in prostate cancer prevention, enhance and perhaps amplify standard treatments. I am certain that tremendous therapeutic advances are out there, we must walk towards them.'

If we are to insist that the idea of diet as a means of preventing or retarding major chronic disease must await the completion of clinical trials, such as those used for medicines designed for the treatment of diseases, the results would be unlikely to became available in time to help anyone aged twenty or over in the year 2008.

Virtually all nutritional and medical researchers who are directly involved with studies on the association between nutrition and major chronic disease would agree on the desirability of such trials, were it practicable to carry them out. So why not? Because unlike trials of medicines, which are to be used for treating fully diagnosed and established diseases in patients, prevention studies must involve vast numbers of individuals who are healthy at the outset, and then monitored for the development of disease over periods of ten to twenty years or even more.

This is because some major chronic diseases, including heart disease and some cancers, take several years, or even decades, to develop to a point at which the disease can be detected and diagnosed. Practical factors, such as the tremendous costs involved and the difficulty of obtaining sufficient volunteers willing to participate over such prolonged periods, render the prospect virtually impossible.

Must we therefore accept that, if the case cannot be proved beyond doubt, then hope of deriving health benefits from foods such as tomatoes should be abandoned? I for one do not, especially as it is only a matter of altering people's eating habits.

CHAPTER 12

Epilogue

It should no longer surprise the reader that consuming a food as ordinary as the tomato can make a very significant contribution to one's health. There is much evidence to suggest that many major chronic diseases, such as cancer and heart disease, could be sparked by the release of free radicals, which are generated in the course of normal everyday metabolism. Because of their structure, these fragments are exceedingly hungry for electrons and waste no time in stealing them from adjacent molecules, thereby destabilising them.

If those molecules happen to be DNA, then a process that leads ultimately to cancer can be started. Because umpteen billions of molecules make up the human body, only a very tiny percentage of such destabilisation on a molecular scale can amount to many thousands of corrupted molecules per second.

Fortunately – otherwise we could not survive – our bodies possess a powerful natural and complex defence mechanism which neutralises the fragments as they arise. Unfortunately, however, the effectiveness of that mechanism tends to diminish with age. Moreover, an ever-increasing number of external factors such as pollution, tobacco smoke and sun exposure also generate free radicals, thereby adding to the problem.

In recent decades, scientists have discovered that our bodies' natural defences are constantly being strengthened by certain constituents present in our food. The extent to which, acting together, they can deal with the growing problem depends on whether we choose to eat a diet which is sufficiently rich in those constituents.

The World Health Organization, international cancer research organisations, the majority of national governmental health agencies and the vast majority of doctors, nutritionists and dieticians all agree: a diet that includes five servings of fruits and vegetables each day reduces the risk of developing cancer and heart disease by up to one third, and helps to gain and maintain a state of good health.

In April 2007, twelve leading companies involved with the manufacture and sale of food and nutritional supplements signed up for a £10 million partnership with the UK Biotechnical and Biological Research Council (BBSRC). This project will provide grants to support further research into the relationship between nutrition and good health. The companies include Cadbury, Glaxo-SmithKline, Nestlé, Unilever and Marks and Spencer.

I have endeavoured to demonstrate, with the help of considerable scientific evidence garnered from the four corners of the globe, that the tomato is a powerful health-promoting companion and bodyguard. Tomatoes are readily available and generally affordable throughout the world. They warrant a place as essential components in our daily five servings of fruits and vegetables. In addition, since eating tomatoes is both pleasurable and harmless, I say let us do it anyway.

To gain the most benefits, an adequate quantity of the tomato's health-promoting constituents must be successfully absorbed into the bloodstream. This, in turn, is influenced among other things by:

1. The variety and growing conditions of the tomato used.

2. The degree of ripeness – the redder the better.
3. The method of food preparation.

The following table is designed to help the reader bypass the complex issues that influence the optimal intake and answer the question: 'How much and how often?'

Incorporate one of the following tomato preparations, together with half to one teaspoonful of virgin olive oil, into your diet daily, or at least three to four times each week.

	Grams	Serving size
Soup	150	One cup
Juice	80	One cup
Cooked whole	300	Two medium tomatoes
Ketchup	50	Two tablespoons
Tomato oleoresin (Lyc-O-Mato)		One capsule
Spaghetti sauce	50	Half cup
Paste	25	Two tablespoons
Purée	50	Two tablespoons
Sauce	50	Quarter cup

Other important elements that make for a healthy lifestyle are well known. Give up smoking, take pleasure in exercise, replace animal fats with vegetable fats, especially olive oil, and enjoy alcohol in moderation and controlled sun exposure.

Storage

According to Jamie Oliver, in *Jamie at Home* (London: Penguin Books, 2007), fresh tomatoes should not be stored in the refrigerator unless fully ripe. After purchase, fresh tomatoes continue to ripen (and increase their health-promoting properties) so long as the temperature is above 12.5°C. Hard, unripe tomatoes placed in the fridge will come out hard and unripe. They keep and taste better when stored in a cool place, out of the sun.

Tomato Recipes

The following recipes are reproduced with permission of the British Tomato Growers Association from their recipe publications.

Hot Stuffed Tomatoes

Serves 4

Ingredients

4 British beef tomatoes
25 g (1 oz) margarine
1 medium onion, peeled and finely chopped
1 small clove garlic, peeled and crushed
2 sticks celery, finely chopped
40 g (1½ oz) fresh wholemeal breadcrumbs
15 ml (1 tbsp) chopped fresh herbs, i.e. basil, oregano, marjoram

1. Stand the tomatoes on their stem ends and slice off the top quarter. Remove the pulp with a small spoon. Stand tomatoes upside down to drain.
2. Melt the margarine in a pan and fry the onion, garlic and celery until soft but not browned. Stir in the breadcrumbs, herbs and tomato pulp. Season well.
3. Fill the tomato cases with the mixture and replace the tops.
4. Cook in the oven at 180 °C (350 °F/gas mark 4) for about twenty minutes. Serve hot.

Classic Tomato Soup

Serves 4

Ingredients

30 ml (2 tbsp) olive oil
2 cloves garlic
900 g (2 lbs) British classic tomatoes, halved
1 small potato, peeled and sliced
300 ml (½ pint) water
5 ml (1 tsp) sugar

1. Lightly oil a roasting tin. Arrange the tomatoes with their cut sides uppermost in the roasting tin. Add the garlic cloves. Season and drizzle over the remaining oil. Roast in the oven at 190 °C (375 °F/gas mark 5) for 30 minutes.
2. Boil the potato in water until tender. Do not drain the water.
3. Skin the tomatoes and the garlic and put the tomato pulp and garlic into a food processor or blender with the cooked potato and potato stock, and blend until smooth.
4. Transfer to a saucepan. Add a little extra vegetable stock or water if the soup is too thick. Stir in the sugar.

Spaghetti Tossed in Mild Chilli and Tomatoes

Serves 4

Ingredients

8 sprays olive oil
1 clove garlic, finely chopped
1 green chilli pepper, deseeded and finely chopped
1 sprig fresh thyme
450 g (1 lb) British classic tomatoes, skinned and halved
15 ml (1 tbsp) capers, drained
250 g (9 oz) spaghetti
350 g (12 oz) British cherry tomatoes
Freshly ground black pepper

1. Preheat the oven to 220 °C (425 °F/gas mark 7).
2. Heat four sprays of olive oil in a saucepan, and sauté garlic and chilli pepper gently for three minutes.
3. Strip the thyme leaves from the stem. Add the skinned tomatoes and thyme leaves to the sauce-pan. Bring slowly to the boil and simmer, uncovered, for about fifteen minutes until the tomatoes are reduced to a fairly thick sauce. Stir in the capers.
4. Meanwhile, cook the spaghetti according to pack instructions.
5. Put the cherry tomatoes in a roasting tin, spray four times with olive oil and roll tomatoes around to coat evenly. Roast tomatoes in the oven for six minutes.
6. Strain the spaghetti and stir in the tomato sauce. Divide between four plates then gently fold in the roasted tomatoes. Add a twist of ground black pepper to each plate of spaghetti and serve immediately.

Tomato Fish Pie

Serves 6

Ingredients

4 small eggs
700 g (1½ lb) potatoes
350 g (12 oz) cod or haddock fillet, skinned and diced
350 g (12 oz) smoked cod or haddock fillet,
   skinned and diced
1 leek, thinly sliced
175 g (6 oz) frozen peas, thawed
150 ml (¼ pint) passata
450 g (1 lb) British classic tomatoes, peeled and
   sliced
30 ml (2 tbsp) chopped parsley
75 g (3 oz) cheddar cheese, grated
15 ml (1 tbsp) milk (optional)

1. Hard-boil eggs for ten minutes. Boil potatoes until tender.
2. Put the fish into a greased 2.3 litre (4 pint) ovenproof casserole. Add the leeks and peas and pour over passata. Arrange a layer of sliced tomatoes on top.
3. Shell the eggs, cut into quarters and place on tomatoes, with yolks uppermost. Season and sprinkle over chopped parsley.
4. Mash the potatoes, and beat in half the cheese and a little milk if necessary to make a creamy consistency.
5. Using a piping bag with a large nozzle, pipe the potato in a lattice pattern on top of the pie. Sprinkle over the remaining grated cheese.
6. Cook in the oven at 190 °C (375 °F/gas mark 5) for 45–55 minutes.

Slow Roast Tomatoes

Try these rich, oily home roast tomatoes instead of sun-dried. They are delicious mixed into salads, pasta and casseroles or chopped into sauces or dressings.

Ingredients

12 British classic or large plum tomatoes
2 tbsp olive oil
1 tsp brown sugar
$\frac{1}{2}$ tsp sea salt flakes
A good twist of ground black pepper

1. Preheat the oven to 190 °C (375 °F/gas mark 5).
2. Cut the tomatoes into quarters and arrange in a single layer in a shallow roasting tin. Toss in the oil, sugar, salt and pepper.
3. Roast in the oven for one-and-a-half to two hours turning from time to time. They are ready when reduced, deep red and just beginning to char. For a 'sun blushed' effect remove the tomatoes from the oven a little earlier.
4. Store in an airtight container and refrigerate for up to two weeks.

Vegetable Moussaka

Serves 6

Ingredients

1 large aubergine
salt
3 large potatoes, peeled and sliced
90 ml (6 tbsp) oil
1 large onion, sliced
900 g (2 lb) British classic tomatoes, peeled and sliced
225 g (8 oz) closed cup mushrooms, sliced
2 large courgettes, thinly sliced
1 red pepper, deseeded and thinly sliced
25 g (1 oz) margarine
25 g (1 oz) flour
300 ml (½ pint) milk
1 medium egg yolk
50 g (2 oz) coarsely grated parmesan cheese

1. Slice aubergine and sprinkle with salt. Leave for half an hour, then drain.
2. Heat 45 ml (3 tbsp) oil in a large frying pan and gently fry the potatoes on both sides for five minutes, until golden brown. Transfer potatoes to a plate and keep warm.
3. Pour the remaining oil into the frying pan and fry the onion till tender. Add the drained aubergines and fry for five minutes.
4. Lightly grease a 2.3 litre (4 pint) casserole dish. Line the casserole dish with half the potatoes. Add half the tomato and aubergine mixture, followed by a layer of

mushrooms, courgettes and red pepper, seasoning each layer. Add the remaining tomato and aubergine mixture and top with the remaining potatoes.

5. Make a white sauce in the usual way, cool slightly, then stir in the egg yolk. Spread the white sauce over the potatoes and sprinkle on the cheese.

6. Cover and cook in the oven at 180 °C (350 °F/ gas mark 4) for one hour. Remove lid and cook for a further half hour.

Tomato and Chickpea Curry

Serves 4

Ingredients

30 ml (2 tbsp) oil
1 onion, sliced
2 cloves garlic, finely chopped
10 ml (2 tsp) ground coriander
5 ml (1 tsp) ground cumin
5 ml (1 tsp) ground turmeric
225 g (8 oz) chestnut mushrooms, halved
190 ml (⅓ pint) vegetable stock
450 g (1 lb) British classic tomatoes, cut into wedges
400 g can chickpeas, drained
45 ml (3 tbsp) chopped fresh coriander

To serve
225 g (8 oz) basmati rice, cooked and drained
Sprig of coriander

1. Heat the oil and cook onion and garlic in a covered pan for about three minutes until soft, then stir in the spices and cook for a minute.
2. Add the remaining ingredients, bring to the boil and simmer gently for about ten minutes.
3. Serve with the cooked basmati rice and garnish with coriander.

Midi Plums with Pesto Crumbs

Serves 4

This dish can be served as an accompaniment to grilled meat or fish, or would make a delicious lunch served with a green salad and crusty bread.

Ingredients

500 g British midi plum or vine tomatoes
15 ml (1 tbsp olive oil)

For the pesto crumbs
15 g basil leaves
15 g pine nuts
15 g freshly grated Parmesan cheese
15 ml (1 tbsp olive oil)
25 g wholemeal breadcrumbs

1. Preheat the oven to 200 °C (400 °F/gas mark 6). Cut the tomatoes in half through the stalk end. Arrange, cut side up, in a shallow baking tin. Bake in the oven for twenty minutes.
2. To make the pesto crumbs: put the basil, pine nuts, Parmesan and olive oil into the bowl of a food processor or liquidiser. Blend to a paste. Add the breadcrumbs and whiz for another minute or two until the breadcrumbs are coated with the pesto mixture.
3. Scatter the crumbs over the tomatoes and drizzle over the tablespoon of olive oil. Return the tomatoes to the oven for another 20–40 minutes. The longer the tomatoes are cooked, the more reduced and intense in flavour they will become.

Spicy Macaroni Cheese

Serves 4

Ingredients

30 ml (2 tbsp) olive oil
1 large onion, finely chopped
1 green pepper, deseeded and chopped
175 g (6 oz) bacon, chopped
125 g (4 oz) closed cup mushrooms, sliced
400 g (14 oz) can chopped peeled tomatoes
60 ml (4 tbsp) tomato purée
30 ml (2 tbsp) Worcestershire sauce
1.25–2.5 ml ($\frac{1}{4}$–$\frac{1}{2}$ tsp) cayenne pepper
198 g (7 oz) can sweetcorn kernels, drained
275 g (10 oz) macaroni, cooked and drained
125 g (4 oz) mature cheddar, grated
25 g (1 oz) dried breadcrumbs

1. Heat the olive oil and cook onion and pepper until just soft. Add the bacon and cook for two minutes. Add the mushrooms and cook for a further minute.
2. Stir in the tomatoes, tomato purée, Worcestershire sauce, cayenne, sweetcorn, and macaroni, then cook over a gentle heat for five minutes.
3. Stir in three-quarters of the cheese. Turn into a warmed heatproof dish.
4. Quickly mix the remaining cheese and breadcrumbs together and sprinkle over the top.
5. Cook under a preheated grill until the cheese has melted and turned golden brown.

Aubergine and Mozzarella Bites

Makes 10–12

It is important to buy an aubergine and two tomatoes that are approximately the same circumference when sliced.

Ingredients

1 aubergine
60 ml (4 tbsp) passata
125 g (4 oz) mozzarella, grated
2 British beef tomatoes, peeled and sliced
10–12 basil leaves
15 ml (1 tbsp) olive oil

1. Slice the aubergine into 1 cm (half-inch) slices. Sprinkle with salt and set aside for half an hour.
2. Rinse, drain and dry the aubergine slices with kitchen paper and arrange on a greased baking tray.
3. Spread a teaspoonful of passata on each aubergine slice and top with mozzarella, tomato slices, seasoning and basil leaves. Drizzle a little oil over each basil leaf.
4. Cook in the oven at 220 °C (425 °F/gas mark 7) for fifteen minutes. Cool for a minute before serving.

Glossary

Describing how the evidence was gathered and interpreted has inevitably involved the use of technical terms. Wherever possible I have tried to simplify or provide an explanation alongside such terms. Some terms or abbreviations that crop up frequently are explained here.

Free radicals and reactive oxygen species
These are molecular or atomic fragments produced during normal metabolism which, if not adequately controlled, can destroy vital tissues by chemical oxidation.

Antioxidants
These are agents that, when present even in very low concentration, can inhibit or delay chemical oxidation.

White Book
The Antioxidants in Tomatoes and their Health Benefits (October 2000) is the title of a document drawn up by scientists from several European countries following a three-year project sponsored by the EU under its Concerted Action Programme. Over the course of the project, four working groups sought answers to the following questions:

1. How do antioxidants present in tomatoes arise, and can they be increased?
2. Does the heating and mechanical processing affect the beneficial constituents of tomatoes or the ease with which they are subsequently absorbed?
3. What have we learned from published studies to date about the protective effects of tomato lycopene against cancer, heart disease and ageing?
4. What are the mechanisms by which tomato lycopene may protect health?

Their document concluded: 'It is clear that tomatoes have a significant contribution to make in terms of public health.'

CHD
Coronary Heart Disease (fully explained in Chapter Four).

Epidemiology studies
Sometimes known as population health studies, these usually involve monitoring very large numbers, often thousands, of volunteers over lengthy periods: five to ten years or more. Comparisons are finally drawn between sub-groups, with the object of identifying present or absent factors that appear to produce beneficial or adverse effects. A classic example was that carried out by Richard Doll and Bradford Hill, which found a proportional relationship between rates of lung cancer and smoking.

Principal References

Chapter 3

K.M. Everson and C.E. McQueen, *American Journal of Health-System Pharmacy*, Vol. 61, pp. 1562–6, 2004

W. Stahl and H. Sies, *Archives of Biochemistry and Biophysics*, Vol. 336, pp. 1–9, 1996

Mendel Friedman, from personal communication with the author

N. O'Kennedy et al, *American Journal of Clinical Nutrition*, Vol. 84, pp. 561–79, 2006

Chapter 4

D. Steinberg et al, *New England Journal of Medicine*, Vol. 320, pp. 915–24, 1989

J.L. Witztum, *Lancet*, Vol. 344, pp. 793–5, 1994

J.T. Salonen and R. Salonen, *Circulation*, Vol. 87, pp. 1156–65, 1993

J.T. Salonen et al, *Circulation*, Vol. 95, pp. 840–5, 1997

M.N. Diaz et al, *New England Journal of Medicine*, Vol. 337, pp. 408–16, 1997

J.T. Salonen et al, *Archives of Toxicology Supplement*, Vol. 20, pp. 249–67, 1998

D.H. O'Leary et al, *New England Journal of Medicine*, Vol. 340, pp.14–22, 1999

T.H. Rissanen et al, *American Journal of Clinical Nutrition*, Vol. 77, pp. 133–8, 2003

A. Duttaroy et al, *Platelets*, Vol. 12, 218–27, 2001

N. O'Kennedy et al, *American Journal of Clinical Nutrition*, Vol. 84, pp. 561–79, 2006

World Health Statistics Quarterly, Vol. 42, pp. 27–149, 1989

E. Giovannucci et al, *Journal of the National Cancer Institute*, Vol. 87, pp. 1767–76, 1995

L. Kohlmeier, *American Journal of Epidemiology*, Vol. 146, pp. 618–26, 1997

A. Keys, *Circulation* supplement, Vol. 41, p. 1, 1970

V.J. Parfitt et al, *European Heart Journal*, Vol. 15, pp. 871, 1994

M. Kristensen, *British Medical Journal*, Vol. 314, pp. 629–33, 1997

E. Gianetti et al, *American Heart Journal*, Vol. 143, p. 467, 2002

T.H. Rissanen et al, *British Journal of Nutrition*, Vol. 85, pp. 749–54, 2001

R. Schmidt et al, *Journal of the Neurological Sciences*, Vol. 152, pp. 15–21, 1997

K. Klipstein-Grobusch et al, *Atherosclosis*, Vol. 148, pp. 49–56, 2000

A.V. Rao and S. Agarwal, *Nutrition Research*, Vol. 18, p. 713, 1998

B. Fuhrman et al, *Biochemical and Biophysical Research Communications*, Vol. 233, pp. 658–62, 1997

L. Arab and S. Steck, *American Journal of Clinical Nutrition* supplement, Vol. 71, pp. 1691S–1695S, 2000

A. Bub et al, *Journal of Nutrition*, Vol. 130, pp. 2200–06, 2000

H.D. Sesso et al, *Nutrition*, Vol. 133, pp. 2336–41, 2003

H.D. Sesso et al, *American Journal of Clinical Nutrition*, Vol. 79, pp. 47–53, 2004

S. Agarwal and A.V. Rao, *Lipids*, Vol. 33, pp. 981–4, 1998

J.L. Witztum, *British Heart Journal* supplement, Vol. 69, pp. S12–18, 1993

P. Reaven et al, *American Journal of Clinical Nutrition*, Vol. 54, pp. 701–06, 1991

P. Reaven et al, *Journal of Clinical Investigation*, Vol. 91, pp. 668–76, 1993

P. Reaven and J.L. Witztum, *The Endocrinologist*, Vol. 5, pp. 44–54, 1995

S. Parthasarathy et al, *Proceedings of the National Academy of Sciences of the United States of America*, Vol. 87, pp. 3894–8, 1991

E.M. Berry et al, *American Journal of Clinical Nutrition*, Vol. 56, pp. 394–403, 1992

H. Esterbauer et al, *Free Radical Biology and Medicine*, Vol. 13, pp. 341–90, 1992

E. Hwang and P. Bowen, *Integrative Cancer Therapies*, Vol. 1, pp. 121–32, 2002

E. Giovannucci and S.K. Clinton, *Journal of the Society for Experimental Biology and Medicine*, Vol. 218, pp. 129–39, 1998

J.K. Campbell et al, *Journal of Nutrition* supplement, Vol. 134, pp. 3486S–3492S, 2004

Chapter 5

G.A. Colditz et al, *American Journal of Clinical Nutrition*, Vol. 41, pp. 32–6, 1985

K.J. Helzlsouer et al, *Cancer Research*, Vol. 49, pp. 6144–8, 1989

P.G. Burney et al, *American Journal of Clinical Nutrition* 1989, 49, 895–900

P.K. Mills et al, *Cancer*, Vol. 64, pp. 598–604, 1989

P. Cook-Mozaffari, *British Journal of Cancer*, Vol. 39, pp. 293–309, 1979

E. Giovannucci et al, *Journal of the National Cancer Institute*, Vol. 87, pp. 1767–76, 1995

P. Gann et al, *Cancer Research*, Vol. 59, pp. 1225–30, 1999

J.M.C. Gutteridge, *British Journal of Biomedical Science*, Vol. 51, pp. 288–95, 1994

A.V. Rao and S. Agarwal, *Nutrition and Cancer*, Vol. 31, pp. 199–203, 1998

E. Giovannucci and S.K. Clinton, *Journal of the Society for Experimental Biology and Medicine*, Vol. 218, pp. 129–39, 1998

E. Giovannucci et al, *Journal of the National Cancer Institute*, Vol. 91, pp. 317–31, 1999

E. Giovannucci, *Journal of the Society for Experimental Biology and Medicine*, Vol. 227, pp. 352–9, 2002

A. Tzonou et al, *International Journal of Cancer*, Vol. 80, pp. 704–08, 1999

Q.Y. Lu et al, *Cancer Epidemiology Biomarkers and Prevention*, Vol. 10, pp. 749–56, 2001

O. Kucuk, *Journal of the Society for Experimental Biology and Medicine*, pp. 227, 881–5, 2002

P. Bowen et al, *Journal of the Society for Experimental Biology and Medicine*, Vol. 227, pp. 886–93, 2002

J.H. Weisburger, *Journal of the Society for Experimental Biology and Medicine*, Vol. 227, pp. 924–7, 2002

C.W. Hadley et al, *Journal of the Society for Experimental Biology and Medicine*, Vol. 227, pp. 869–80, 2002

E. Hwang and P. Bowen, *Integrative Cancer Therapies*, Vol. 1, pp. 121–32, 2002

J.K. Campbell et al, *Journal of Nutrition*, Vol. 134, pp. 3486S–3492S, 2004

Chapter 6

E. Giovannucci et al, *Journal of the National Cancer Institute*, Vol. 87, pp. 1767–76, 1995

J. Gartner et al, *American Journal of Clinical Nutrition*, Vol. 66, pp. 116–22, 1997

M. Porrini, First International Conference on Health Benefits of Lycopene, Washington, DC, 2 April 2003

J.M. Fielding, *Asian Pacific Journal of Clinical Nutrition*, Vol. 14, pp. 131–6, 2005

S.K. Clinton, *Nutrition Reviews*, Vol. 56, pp. 35–51, 1998

W. Stahl and H. Sies, *Journal of Nutrition*, Vol. 122, pp. 2161–6, 1992

F. Khachik, *Experimental Biology and Medicine*, Vol. 227, pp. 845–51, 2002

P. Trumbo, *Journal of Nutrition*, Vol. 135, pp. 2023S, 2005

McClaren, *Sight and Life Newsletter*, No. 2, p. 18, 2000

K.M. Everson and C.E. McQueen, *American Journal of Health-System Pharmacy*, Vol. 61, p. 1562–6, 2004

S. Agarwal and A.V. Rao, *Lipids*, Vol. 33, pp. 981–4, 1998

The Antioxidants in Tomatoes and their Health Benefits (*White Book*), EU Concerted Action Programme, October 2000

R. Peto et al, *Nature*, Vol. 290, pp. 201–08, 1981

S. Astley, *Journal of Nutrition*, Vol. 135, pp. 2027–8, 2005

D.W. Voskvil, *Cancer Epidemiology Biomarkers and Prevention*, Vol. 14, pp. 195–203, 2005

Mucci et al, *British Journal of Urology International*, Vol. 87, pp. 814–20, 2001

V. Siler et al, *FASEB Journal*, Vol. 18, pp. 1019–21, 2004

P. Boyle et al, *Urologic Clinics of North America*, Vol. 30, pp. 209–17, 2003

O. Kucuk, *Cancer Epidemiology Biomarkers and Prevention*, Vol. 10, pp. 861–8, 2001

J. Levy et al, *Nutrition and Cancer*, Vol. 24, pp. 257–66, 1995

B. Fuhrman et al, *Biochemical and Biophysical Research Communications*, Vol. 223, pp. 658–62, 1997

Chapter 7

J.B. Sharma, *International Journal of Gynecology and Obstetrics*, Vol. 94, pp. 23–7, 2006, and *International Journal of Gynecology and Obstetrics*, Vol. 81, pp. 257–62, 2003 (the study)

J.A. Mares and S.M. Moeller, *American Journal of Clinical Nutrition*, Vol. 83, pp. 733–4, 2006

R. van Leewen et al, *Journal of the American Medical Association*, Vol, 294, pp. 3101–07, 2005

F. Khachik, *Experimental Biology and Medicine*, Vol. 227, pp. 845–51, 2002

L.G. Rao, *Endocrinology Rounds*, St Michael's Hospital, Toronto, 2005

A. Zini, *International Journal of Andrology*, Vol. 16, p. 183, 1993

Gupta, *Heinz Nutritional Newsletter*, April 2003, p. 3

N.K. Mohatny, *Indian Journal of Urology*, Vol. 56, p. 102, 2001

W. Stahl, *Journal of Nutrition*, Vol. 131, pp. 1449–51, 2001

L.G. Rao et al, *Journal of Medicinal Food*, Vol. 6, pp. 69–78, 2003

J.P. Cesarini et al, *Photodermatology, Photoimmunology and Photomedicine*, Vol. 19, pp. 182–9, 2003

A.O. Aust, *International Journal for Vitamin and Nutrition Research*, Vol. 75, pp. 54–60, 2005

M. Andreassi, *Journal of the European Academy of Dermatology and Venereology*, Vol. 18, pp. 52–5, 2004

S. Francheschi et al, *International Journal of Cancer*, Vol. 59, p. 81, 1994

J. Levy et al, *Nutrition and Cancer*, Vol. 24, pp. 257–66, 1995

H. Sies et al, *Annals of the New York Academy of Sciences*, Vol. 669, pp. 7–20, 1992

J.A. Yuan et al, *Cancer Epidemiology Biomarkers and Prevention*, Vol. 13, pp. 1772–80, 2004

Y. Ito, *Asian Pacific Journal of Cancer Prevention*, Vol. 6, pp. 10–15, 2005

A. Aguda, *European Journal of Cancer*, Vol. 33, pp. 1256–61, 1997

S. Darby, *British Journal of Cancer*, Vol. 84, pp. 728–35, 2001

Y. Ito, *Cancer Science*, Vol. 94, pp. 57–63, 2003

T. Coyne et al, *American Journal of Clinical Nutrition*, Vol. 24, pp. 448–55, 2005

J. Wood, *Journal of the American College of Nutrition*, Vol. 24, pp. 448–55, 2005

I. Neuman, *Allergy*, Vol. 55, p. 1184, 2000

D.J. Pattison et al, *American Journal of Clinical Nutrition*, Vol. 82, pp. 451–5, 2005

A. Duttaroy et al, *Platelets*, Vol. 12, pp. 218–27, 2001

Index

A

M

N

O

R

S

T